INTERSTITIAL CYSTITIS

COOKBOOK

DR. ROWAN VITALIS

INTERSTITIAL CYSTITIS COOKBOOK

DR. ROWAN VITALIS

COPYRIGHT

© 2025 by Dr. Rowan Vitalis

All rights reserved.

No part of this book may be reproduced, distributed, or transmitted in any form or by any means, including photocopying, recording, or other electronic or mechanical methods, without prior written permission from the publisher, except in the case of brief quotations used in book reviews or other permitted uses under copyright law.

DISCLAIMER

The information provided in this cookbook is intended for educational and informational purposes only. The recipes and dietary advice are not intended to be a substitute for professional medical advice.

While the recipes in this book are designed to be healthy and nutritious, every individual is different, and it is important to consult with your doctor or a registered dietitian before making any significant changes to your diet.

The author and publisher of this cookbook do not assume any responsibility for any adverse reactions, health problems, or side effects that may occur as a result of following the information or recipes contained in this book.

By using this cookbook, you agree to release the author and publisher from any liability or responsibility for any adverse reactions, health problems, or side effects that may occur as a result of following the information or recipes contained herein.

TABLE OF CONTENT

Introduction

   How Diet Influences Interstitial Cystitis (IC/BPS)

   Core Principles of the IC Diet

Chapter 1: Bladder-Friendly Foods and Ingredients

   Making Smart Substitutions for Common Bladder Irritants

   Shopping Tips for Managing Interstitial Cystitis (IC)

Chapter 3: IC-Friendly Recipes

BREAKFAST RECIPES

1. Oatmeal with Banana and Almond Butter
2. Coconut Yogurt Parfait with Melon and Blueberries
3. Scrambled Eggs with Spinach and Zucchini
4. Chia Seed Pudding with Pear and Coconut Flakes
5. Rice Pudding with Cinnamon and Pears
6. Sweet Potato Hash with Turkey Sausage
7. Quinoa and Blueberry Breakfast Bowl
8. Coconut Flour Pancakes with Maple Syrup
9. Avocado Toast with Hemp Seeds
10. Apple Cinnamon Smoothie
11. Rice Cake with Almond Butter and Strawberries
12. Vegetable Omelet with Zucchini and Carrot
13. Non-Dairy Banana Smoothie
14. Baked Oats with Blueberries and Cinnamon
15. Coconut Chia Pudding with Kiwi
16. Zucchini Noodles with Avocado Pesto

17. Oatmeal with Pear and Cinnamon

18. Pineapple Coconut Smoothie

19. Buckwheat Pancakes with Maple Syrup

20. Coconut and Blueberry Muffins

LUNCH RECIPES

21. Chicken Salad with Mixed Greens

22. Quinoa Bowl with Roasted Veggies

23. Rice and Chicken Stir-Fry

24. Turkey and Avocado Lettuce Wraps

25. Grilled Salmon with Steamed Asparagus

26. Zucchini Noodles with Chicken and Olive Oil

27. Sweet Potato and Black Bean Bowl

28. Quinoa and Veggie Stuffed Sweet Potatoes

29. Grilled Chicken with Brown Rice and Green Beans

30. Vegetable Soup with Rice

31. Chicken and Spinach Salad with Olive Oil Dressing

32. Lentil Salad with Cucumber and Tomatoes

33. Chicken and Sweet Potato Stew

34. Rice and Veggie Casserole

35. Cucumber and Avocado Sushi Rolls

36. Turkey and Cucumber Salad

37. Egg Salad with Avocado and Spinach

38. Grilled Veggie Wrap with Hummus

39. Baked Chicken with Roasted Carrots and Quinoa

40. Coconut Milk Chicken Soup

DINNER RECIPES

41. Baked Salmon with Sweet Potatoes and Steamed Broccoli

42. Turkey Meatballs with Brown Rice and Squash

43. Vegetable Soup with Carrots, Zucchini, and Celery

44. Chicken and Quinoa Stir Fry with Spinach

45. Grilled Chicken with Roasted Vegetables

46. Baked Cod with Steamed Carrots and Sweet Potatoes

47. Chicken and Sweet Potato Stew

48. Stuffed Yellow Squash with Quinoa and Turkey

49. Herb Grilled Salmon with Brown Rice

50. Vegetable Stir Fry with Tofu and Brown Rice

51. Grilled Chicken with Avocado and Cucumber Salad

52. Baked Chicken with Steamed Asparagus and Quinoa

53. Quinoa and Vegetable Patties

54. Lentil Soup with Carrots and Zucchini

55. Baked Turkey with Roasted Carrots and Green Beans

56. Zucchini Noodles with Grilled Chicken and Olive Oil

57. Chicken and Avocado Lettuce Wraps

58. Grilled Veggie Skewers with Brown Rice

59. Pork Tenderloin with Roasted Carrots and Spinach

60. Coconut Milk Chicken Curry with Steamed Vegetables

SNACK RECIPES

61. Homemade Granola Bars

62. Rice Cakes with Avocado

63. Non-Dairy Yogurt Parfait

64. Carrot and Cucumber Sticks with Hummus

65. Baked Apple Chips

66. Banana and Almond Butter Bites

67. Zucchini Chips

68. Coconut Chia Pudding

69. Rice Cake with Almond Butter and Pear Slices

70. Apple Slices with Almond Butter

71. Oatmeal Energy Balls

72. Quinoa Salad Cups

73. Coconut Yogurt with Blueberries

74. Cucumber and Avocado Slices

75. Steamed Sweet Potato Slices

76. Baked Sweet Potato Fries

77. Peach Chia Smoothie

78. Hummus and Rice Crackers

79. Coconut Flake Energy Balls

80. Avocado Smoothie

Chapter 4: 14-Day Meal Plan for IC Patients

Chapter 5: Caring for a Loved One with IC — Practical Support for Family Members and Caregivers

Helping with Food Choices and Meal Prep for Someone Living with Interstitial Cystitis

Dining Out and Social Gatherings: How to Navigate Restaurants and Events While Following the IC Diet

Conclusion

Introduction

Interstitial Cystitis, often referred to as **Bladder Pain Syndrome**, is a complex, long-term condition that affects people in ways that can't always be seen from the outside. For many, it means living with persistent bladder discomfort, a pressing need to urinate frequently—even when the bladder isn't full—and sharp pain that can interrupt sleep, make travel difficult, and disrupt work or social life without warning.

The cause isn't fully known, which adds another layer of frustration. Researchers suspect that it may involve inflammation of the bladder lining, nerve sensitivity, and problems in the way the bladder holds and signals fluid. What's certain is that no two experiences with this condition are the same. Symptoms show up differently from person to person, and even from day to day.

People living with IC often report pain ranging from a dull ache to intense burning or pressure in the lower abdomen or pelvic region. That pain may come and go—or show up suddenly after certain meals, activities, or stressors. Urgency and frequency are common too. Some people feel like they need to go to the bathroom every 20 minutes, sometimes even waking up throughout the night to do so. Others feel pain while urinating or just after, with a sensation of pressure that makes relaxing nearly impossible. It's a condition that doesn't just affect the bladder—it touches every part of life.

Living with IC can be draining in every sense of the word. The constant discomfort, the unpredictability of flare-ups, the way meals become stressful instead of joyful—it can all feel like too much. And when symptoms spike without warning, people often feel isolated, misunderstood, or even blamed for something completely outside their control.

The good news? There's one area where you can take back some control: what you eat.

Over time, many people with IC have discovered that the foods they consume can either help calm the bladder—or aggravate it. While no single diet works for everyone, there are ingredients that are more bladder-friendly and others that are more likely to cause irritation. This doesn't mean you're stuck with bland, repetitive meals. Quite the opposite. With the right approach, your meals can be nourishing, satisfying, and designed to support comfort.

That's exactly why this cookbook exists.

Inside these pages, you'll find recipes created specifically for people managing IC. Every meal is built around foods that are known to be gentle on the bladder. You'll also find helpful insights to guide your food choices—not in a rigid or judgmental way, but in a way that empowers you to make decisions that support your health.

These recipes were created not only to nourish your body but also to help ease the daily burden of this condition. The goal isn't perfection—it's progress. Small, thoughtful shifts in what you eat can make a real difference over time, especially when flare-ups start to lessen and energy returns. You'll begin to feel more confident in your meals and more connected to your own healing.

This book was also created with caregivers and family members in mind. If someone you care about has IC, you might feel helpless watching them struggle to find meals that don't make things worse. It can be overwhelming to navigate dietary changes together, especially when typical cookbooks don't take IC into account. That's where this guide comes in. It gives you the tools to prepare meals that truly support their comfort, without sacrificing taste or nutrition.

Even if you haven't been diagnosed with IC but are trying to minimize your risk or support a sensitive bladder, this cookbook can still be an essential part of your kitchen. Following a gentle, anti-inflammatory approach to eating has benefits far beyond the bladder. It can help balance your digestion, improve your sleep, and promote a more stable mood—because when the body is less inflamed, it functions better as a whole.

The information here isn't based on trends or internet myths. It's grounded in current research, real-life experience, and a practical understanding of how food interacts with the bladder. You won't find general advice or vague meal plans. Every page has been carefully designed to offer real help, with recipes that make it easier to live well.

Instead of offering strict rules, this book provides tools. You'll be able to build your own version of a bladder-friendly diet—one that's flexible enough for daily life and nourishing enough to support healing. The recipes here are meant to be part of a lifestyle that works with your body, not against it.

Whether you're looking for ideas to make meals less stressful, searching for support during a flare, or simply trying to feel more comfortable day to day, this cookbook is for you. You'll find meals that are gentle but never boring, ingredients that are carefully chosen for your needs, and guidance that removes the guesswork from your kitchen.

Eating with IC doesn't have to feel like giving something up. With the right knowledge and the right ingredients, it becomes an opportunity to care for your body in a way that feels good—physically, emotionally, and mentally.

How Diet Influences Interstitial Cystitis (IC/BPS)

What you eat plays a powerful role in how your bladder feels—especially when you're living with Interstitial Cystitis (IC) or Bladder Pain Syndrome (BPS). Although the root cause of IC/BPS is still not fully understood, one thing is clear for many people: certain foods can trigger symptoms, while others seem to calm them. This makes diet a valuable tool in your IC management strategy.

The bladder lining in those with IC tends to be more reactive than normal, meaning it can become irritated by ingredients or compounds that wouldn't bother someone without the condition. As a result, flare-ups of pain, urgency, and frequent urination are often directly linked to dietary choices.

The upside? Changing the way you eat—by minimizing irritants and adding in more soothing options—can bring real relief. Even small adjustments can lead to a noticeable improvement in your comfort and give you a greater sense of control over your symptoms.

Common Foods That Can Trigger IC Flare-Ups

Certain foods and drinks have a well-earned reputation for irritating the bladder. These aren't just uncomfortable—they can cause inflammation or spark an overactive immune response, leading to flare-ups that disrupt your daily life. Knowing which ingredients to watch out for is the first step in reducing these episodes.

Here are some of the most common dietary irritants for those with IC:

- **Acidic Fruits and Foods:** Oranges, lemons, limes, grapefruit, tomatoes, and anything with high acidity can aggravate the bladder. These foods often lead to stinging, pain, or an increase in urgency.
- **Caffeinated Drinks:** Coffee, regular tea, energy drinks, and colas don't just wake you up—they also stimulate the bladder and act as diuretics, making you need to urinate more often and urgently.
- **Spicy Foods:** Hot peppers, chili powder, curry, and other spicy seasonings can inflame the sensitive bladder lining, setting off a chain reaction of discomfort.
- **Alcoholic Beverages:** Wine, beer, and cocktails are frequent triggers. Alcohol can both irritate the bladder and dehydrate the body, compounding the problem by increasing frequency.

- **Artificial Sweeteners:** Sugar substitutes like aspartame, saccharin, and sucralose can cause issues for many people with IC. They're commonly found in diet sodas, sugar-free gum, and low-calorie snacks, making them easy to overlook.

Cutting out or reducing these bladder offenders can make a huge difference. At first, it might feel restrictive—but over time, you'll likely find that avoiding them gives you much more freedom and peace of mind.

Foods That Soothe and Support Bladder Health

These are the ones that are gentle, nourishing, and packed with anti-inflammatory properties. Adding more of these items into your diet can help reduce irritation and support healing.

Here's a list of bladder-friendly options to focus on:

- **Low-Acid Fruits:** Not all fruit is off-limits. Apples, pears, blueberries, and melons like cantaloupe and watermelon offer fiber, antioxidants, and natural sweetness—without provoking symptoms.
- **Lean Protein:** Skinless chicken, turkey, and mild fish such as cod or salmon are good choices. These protein sources are filling and nutritious, and they're less likely to trigger inflammation than red meats or processed options.
- **Whole Grains:** Brown rice, quinoa, oats, and other minimally processed grains provide steady energy and promote digestive health—both of which contribute to bladder stability.
- **Herbal Teas:** Instead of reaching for caffeinated beverages, try herbal teas such as chamomile, peppermint, or ginger. They can have calming effects on both your nervous system and your bladder.
- **Cooked Vegetables:** Gentle veggies like zucchini, sweet potatoes, carrots, cucumbers, spinach, and kale are excellent. Steaming or roasting makes them even easier to digest, which can minimize irritation.

- **Healthy Fats:** Incorporating anti-inflammatory fats like olive oil, avocado, and ground flaxseeds helps the body reduce inflammation over time—including in the bladder.

The more you build meals around these calming foods, the easier it becomes to manage symptoms. They're not just safer choices—they actively contribute to your long-term bladder healing.

Building a Balanced Diet That Works for You

Managing IC/BPS isn't just about cutting out irritants or sticking to a list of "safe" foods. It's about creating a well-rounded diet that works with your body. Because everyone with IC experiences symptoms differently, your personal triggers and tolerances may not look exactly like someone else's.

That said, the foundation of an IC-friendly diet remains the same: focus on whole, unprocessed foods that reduce inflammation and are easy on your bladder. Think of it as building meals from the inside out—choosing ingredients that support healing while avoiding those that may set you back.

For example:
- Omega-3s found in foods like salmon, flaxseeds, and chia seeds help calm the immune system and reduce inflammation at a cellular level.
- Whole grains such as quinoa or oatmeal offer a steady source of energy without the blood sugar spikes or digestive stress that can aggravate IC symptoms.
- Swapping soda for a cooling herbal tea isn't just a good move for your bladder—it supports hydration and calm from the inside out.

This cookbook is designed to guide you toward meals and snacks that are as enjoyable as they are bladder-friendly. In chapter three of the book, you'll find recipes that make it easier to manage symptoms, reduce the likelihood of flare-ups, and support healing every day.

Core Principles of the IC Diet

The Interstitial Cystitis (IC) diet is built around one central idea: reduce irritation, support healing. At its core, this approach focuses on avoiding foods and drinks that aggravate the bladder, while encouraging gentle, nourishing options that calm inflammation and support your overall well-being.

These principles aren't just about managing symptoms—they're about creating a lifestyle that makes living with IC/BPS more comfortable and balanced.

A Gentle Approach to Food

The philosophy behind the IC diet is simple: by choosing soothing, bladder-friendly foods, you can help reduce flare-ups without giving up flavor or nutrition. Learning the basics of this diet gives you the tools to make thoughtful choices that support your body and help ease discomfort.

Avoiding Bladder Irritants

The first key step in the IC diet is identifying and avoiding foods that are known to irritate the bladder. This might take some adjustment, but cutting out these triggers can lead to noticeable relief.

Again, here are some of the most common culprits:

- **Acidic Foods:** Citrus fruits (like oranges, lemons, grapefruit), tomatoes, and tomato-based sauces can be harsh on the bladder lining. Even seemingly healthy options like orange juice or a spicy marinara sauce may cause flare-ups in sensitive individuals.

- **Spicy Foods:** Hot peppers, chili, and meals seasoned with cayenne, curry, or hot sauce can increase bladder sensitivity. While they may be flavorful, avoiding spicy ingredients is important for keeping symptoms in check.

- **Caffeine:** Found in coffee, many teas, energy drinks, and sodas, caffeine is a stimulant that can irritate the bladder and increase the urgency to urinate. Try replacing it with herbal teas that are gentler on the system.

- **Alcohol:** Beer, wine, cocktails, and spirits can all aggravate the bladder. Not only is alcohol a diuretic—meaning it increases urination—but it also often contains acids and artificial additives that can further irritate sensitive tissues.

- **Processed Foods:** Packaged snacks, canned soups, instant meals, and fast food often contain preservatives, artificial sweeteners, and other chemicals that can trigger bladder symptoms. Reducing processed foods can make a big difference in how you feel.

Embracing Soothing, Anti-Inflammatory Foods

Just as important as avoiding irritants is the inclusion of healing, calming foods. These choices are typically mild, anti-inflammatory, and easy on the bladder.

- **Non-Acidic Fruits:** Apples, pears, and melons like cantaloupe and watermelon are great options. They offer fiber, vitamins, and natural sweetness without the sting of citrus.

- **Lean Proteins:** Chicken, turkey, and non-acidic fish like salmon or cod are excellent protein sources that support tissue repair and overall health without aggravating the bladder.

- **Whole Grains:** Brown rice, oats, quinoa, and other whole grains are rich in fiber and nutrients. They provide long-lasting energy and are generally well tolerated by those with IC.

- **Vegetables:** Cooked, non-acidic vegetables like zucchini, carrots, sweet potatoes, cucumbers, and leafy greens (like spinach and kale) are packed with antioxidants and vitamins. These support healing and are typically gentle on the bladder.

- **Healthy Fats:** Fats from avocados, olive oil, flaxseeds, and other natural sources can help reduce inflammation throughout the body. These beneficial fats are great for your overall health and can be an important part of a balanced, IC-friendly diet.

Finding Balance for Symptom Relief

Creating a balanced diet is essential—not just one that avoids triggers, but one that leaves you feeling satisfied and nourished. Strive to include a good mix of:

- Lean proteins
- Whole grains
- Healthy fats
- Bladder-friendly fruits and vegetables

Hydration is also key. Water is the best choice for keeping your bladder functioning well and flushing out irritants. Herbal teas like chamomile or ginger can be soothing alternatives to caffeinated beverages.

Personalization Is Everything

One of the most important things to understand about the IC diet is that it's not one-size-fits-all. While many foods are commonly tolerated or commonly avoided, everyone's body is different.

Keeping a food journal can help you identify your personal triggers and patterns. Over time, you'll be able to adjust your diet to reflect what truly works for you.

In Summary

The foundation of the IC diet is about avoiding irritants—like acidic fruits, spicy foods, caffeine, alcohol, and processed meals—**while choosing gentle, nourishing foods that soothe the bladder,** such as non-acidic fruits, lean proteins, whole grains, and anti-inflammatory vegetables.

By listening to your body and adjusting your choices, you can create a diet that not only reduces IC symptoms but also supports your overall health. With consistency, this approach can empower you to feel more in control and live with greater comfort and ease.

Chapter 1: Bladder-Friendly Foods and Ingredients

Making Smart Substitutions for Common Bladder Irritants

When adhering to a bladder-friendly diet for managing Interstitial Cystitis (IC), making thoughtful substitutions can significantly improve your meals, ensuring they remain both flavorful and gentle on your bladder. Many typical ingredients commonly found in everyday cooking can irritate the bladder or aggravate symptoms. Thankfully, there are many tasty and easy alternatives available that provide the same texture and flavor while offering soothing benefits. The key to success lies in replacing irritants with gentler choices that help nourish your body and safeguard your bladder.

Below are several common bladder irritants, along with their bladder-friendly substitutes:

1. Dairy Products

Dairy products such as milk, cheese, and yogurt can often be triggers for individuals dealing with IC due to their acidic nature, high-fat content, and tendency to promote mucus production, all of which can aggravate bladder discomfort. Fortunately, several dairy-free alternatives can easily be incorporated into your meals.

- **Coconut Milk and Almond Milk:** These plant-based milks serve as excellent replacements for cow's milk. Coconut milk is creamy and mild in flavor, making it ideal for smoothies, soups, and sauces. Almond milk, on the other hand, is light and versatile, perfect for use in baking, with cereal, or even as a base for coffee. Both options are naturally low in acidity and gentle on the bladder.

- **Coconut Yogurt and Almond Yogurt:** If you're a yogurt fan, try substituting regular dairy yogurt with coconut or almond yogurt. These dairy-free alternatives are typically made from coconut or almond milk and are much less likely to cause irritation. Available in a variety of flavors, they can be enjoyed on their own, in parfaits, or added to smoothies, topped with a drizzle of honey or fresh fruits.

- **Dairy-Free Cheeses:** There are now many dairy-free cheeses made from coconut, cashews, or almonds. These cheeses can be used in recipes like pizzas, sandwiches, or casseroles. Look for products that are low in additives and preservatives to ensure they remain easy on the bladder.

2. Tomatoes

Tomatoes, particularly when raw or used in sauces, can be highly acidic and may irritate the bladder. While you might miss their tangy flavor, there are simple ways to recreate similar tastes without causing discomfort.

- **Mild Vegetable-Based Sauces:** Instead of using tomato-based sauces, consider making vegetable-based sauces using ingredients like carrots, zucchini, or bell peppers. These vegetables are naturally sweet and mild, and when cooked down into a sauce, they provide a flavorful and satisfying base for pasta, rice, or grain dishes.

  For example, a zucchini and carrot sauce can be pureed with garlic and olive oil to create a rich, creamy texture that works wonderfully as a pasta topping. Roasted bell peppers combined with garlic and olive oil can also create a mild, slightly sweet sauce that pairs well with a variety of dishes.

- **Pumpkin Puree:** Pumpkin puree is another fantastic substitute for tomatoes in soups and sauces. It is naturally sweet and creamy, adding a rich texture without causing irritation. You can also use pumpkin puree in baked goods like muffins and pancakes for a comforting, nutrient-dense addition.

- **Butternut Squash:** Similar to pumpkin, butternut squash has a smooth, sweet flavor when cooked and blended. It can be used as a substitute for tomatoes in soups, stews, or sauces. Roasting the squash first will bring out its natural sweetness and add depth to your dishes.

3. Spices and Seasonings

Spicy seasonings such as cayenne pepper, hot peppers, and chili powder can trigger flare-ups for individuals with IC. While you don't have to sacrifice flavor in your cooking, it is important to opt for milder seasonings that are gentler on the bladder.

- **Herbs Instead of Spicy Seasonings:** Rather than reaching for hot spices like chili or cayenne pepper, experiment with bladder-friendly herbs like basil, oregano, parsley, thyme, and dill. These herbs add robust flavor without causing irritation. Whether fresh or dried, these herbs can elevate the taste of your dishes without the heat.

- **Ginger and Turmeric:** For a touch of warming spice, ginger and turmeric make excellent alternatives. Ginger provides a mild, soothing heat that supports digestion and reduces inflammation, while turmeric offers an earthy flavor along with its powerful anti-inflammatory properties. Both spices can be incorporated into soups, teas, and marinades.

- **Garlic and Onion:** While raw onions can be an irritant for some people, cooked onions and garlic are typically well-tolerated in moderation. Sautéing garlic in olive oil or using roasted onions can bring out their natural sweetness and flavor without the harsh bite of raw onions.

4. Caffeine and Alcohol

Caffeine and alcohol are known bladder irritants, as they can increase urinary frequency and contribute to discomfort. Fortunately, there are plenty of non-caffeinated, alcohol-free beverages that provide a soothing experience.

- **Herbal Teas:** Instead of coffee or caffeinated tea, consider sipping on herbal teas like chamomile, peppermint, or ginger. These teas are calming and their natural properties can help ease bladder discomfort. Chamomile tea, for example, has been used for centuries to help with inflammation and promote relaxation.

- **Decaf Coffee and Tea:** If you miss the taste of coffee or regular tea, try their decaffeinated versions. These options are gentler on the bladder while still offering the warmth and ritual of your favorite morning drink.

- **Fruit-Infused Water:** For a refreshing and hydrating alternative, infuse your water with bladder-friendly fruits like cucumber, melon, or berries. You can also infuse water with herbs like mint to add a subtle, natural flavor, making it more enjoyable to stay hydrated without the irritation of caffeinated or alcoholic beverages.

5. Gluten and Processed Grains

Gluten, found in wheat and many processed grains, can be an irritant for some individuals with IC. If you find that gluten worsens your symptoms, there are numerous gluten-free alternatives that still provide essential nutrients.

- **Gluten-Free Grains:** Instead of wheat-based products, try quinoa, brown rice, oats, or amaranth. These grains are naturally gluten-free and provide fiber, protein, and other nutrients to support overall health.

- **Almond Flour and Coconut Flour:** When baking, substitute regular flour with almond flour or coconut flour. These gluten-free alternatives are perfect for making IC-friendly baked goods, such as muffins, pancakes, and cookies, without causing irritation.

- **Rice Noodles or Zucchini Noodles:** For pasta dishes, you can replace traditional pasta with rice noodles or zucchini noodles (often called "zoodles"). These options are gluten-free and provide a satisfying alternative to wheat-based pasta while being gentle on the bladder.

6. Processed and Packaged Foods

Many processed and packaged foods contain artificial preservatives, sweeteners, and additives that can irritate the bladder. By choosing whole foods and cooking from scratch, you can avoid these potential irritants.

- **Homemade Snacks:** Instead of packaged chips or snacks, consider making your own IC-friendly versions at home. For example, you can make baked sweet potato chips or zucchini chips by slicing the vegetables and baking them with a drizzle of olive oil and a pinch of salt.

- **Whole, Fresh Ingredients:** Whenever possible, use fresh, whole ingredients to prepare your meals. This allows you to have complete control over the ingredients, ensuring that your food is free from artificial additives and preservatives.

By making these substitutions, you can enjoy delicious meals that are safe for your bladder while still satisfying your taste buds. Finding alternatives for common irritants can empower you to stick to your diet and manage your IC symptoms effectively without feeling restricted. With a little creativity, you can continue enjoying flavorful meals that support bladder health and overall well-being.

Shopping Tips for Managing Interstitial Cystitis (IC)

Navigating the grocery store when you have Interstitial Cystitis (IC) can feel overwhelming. With so many food choices, many of which may contain bladder-irritating ingredients, it's challenging to stick to a diet that promotes bladder health. However, with a little direction, shopping for bladder-friendly foods can become a much easier and more intuitive experience. By learning what to look for and what to avoid, you can make informed decisions that not only help manage your IC symptoms but also support overall bladder health.

Here are some practical tips that will help you shop confidently for foods that are IC-friendly:

1. Opt for Whole, Fresh Foods

The cornerstone of an IC-friendly diet is fresh, whole foods, as close to their natural state as possible. These foods tend to be less processed and free of preservatives, artificial additives, and chemicals that can irritate the bladder.

- **Stick to the Perimeter of the Store:** Most grocery stores have fresh produce, meats, and dairy (or dairy alternatives) located along the perimeter. Focus on filling your cart with these items, such as fresh fruits, vegetables, lean meats, and whole grains. These foods provide the foundation for a nourishing and healing diet.

- **Choose Fresh over Canned:** Whenever possible, opt for fresh fruits and vegetables rather than canned versions. Canned foods often contain added sodium, preservatives, and sometimes citric acid, all of which can irritate the bladder. If you must buy canned goods, look for options labeled "no added salt" or "no added sugar," and ensure the ingredient list is as minimal as possible.

2. Carefully Read Food Labels

One of the most critical skills when shopping for an IC-friendly diet is learning how to read food labels effectively. Many packaged foods contain hidden irritants that could trigger IC flare-ups.

- **Look for Hidden Irritants:** Pay close attention to ingredients such as citrus, spices, vinegar, and artificial sweeteners (like aspartame, sucralose, and saccharin). These are common sources of bladder irritation.

- **Avoid Preservatives and Additives:** Stay away from foods with long ingredient lists full of preservatives, artificial colors, and flavor enhancers like monosodium glutamate (MSG). These are commonly found in processed snacks, sauces, and ready-made meals.

- **Check for Dairy, Gluten, and Soy:** If you're sensitive to dairy, gluten, or soy, always check the labels for these ingredients. Many people with IC find that these can aggravate their symptoms. Look for dairy-free, gluten-free, and soy-free products if these are triggers for you.

- **Understand Serving Sizes:** Sometimes, the serving size on packaged foods is much smaller than what you might typically eat. Be sure to account for this when reviewing the ingredient list and nutritional information. Even a seemingly harmless ingredient can impact your symptoms if consumed in larger amounts.

3. Seek IC-Friendly Substitutes

A key strategy in managing IC symptoms is replacing potential irritants with safer alternatives. Many common ingredients can be swapped for options that provide similar textures and flavors without irritating the bladder.

- **Dairy Substitutes:** Look for plant-based milks like almond, coconut, or oat milk, along with dairy-free cheeses and yogurts. Many stores offer a variety of options made from almonds, cashews, coconut, or soy (if soy is not a trigger). These alternatives are often fortified with calcium and vitamins, providing the same nutritional benefits as dairy without the irritation.

- **Gluten-Free Products:** If gluten is a trigger for your IC, seek out products labeled "gluten-free." Many stores offer a wide selection of gluten-free breads, pastas, crackers, and snacks made from alternative grains like rice, quinoa, and oats. Just be cautious of gluten-free processed foods, as they may still contain other irritants like sugar and preservatives.

- **Low-Acid Sauces:** When choosing sauces, look for vegetable-based alternatives to tomato-based ones. If you enjoy pasta sauces or pizza, try tomato-free options or make your own simple olive oil and garlic sauce or a pureed vegetable sauce using mild ingredients like zucchini, carrots, or butternut squash.

4. Choose Gentle and Soothing Ingredients

As you shop, aim to incorporate ingredients that are known for being gentle on the bladder. These foods can help reduce inflammation, soothe irritation, and promote bladder calmness. Focus on foods with anti-inflammatory properties and those that support digestion and hydration.

- **Hydrating Fruits and Vegetables:** Watermelon, cantaloupe, cucumbers, and zucchini are excellent choices for staying hydrated and soothing the bladder. These foods are low in acidity and high in water content, which helps flush the bladder and keep it calm.

- **Non-Acidic, Non-Spicy Foods:** Avoid foods high in acid or spice. Opt for milder vegetables like spinach, carrots, sweet potatoes, and squash, which are gentler on the bladder. Fresh herbs like basil, oregano, and parsley can add flavor without the heat.

- **Healthy Fats:** Incorporate healthy fats from sources like olive oil, avocados, and flaxseeds. These fats provide anti-inflammatory benefits and are less likely to irritate the bladder compared to fats like butter or processed oils.

5. Focus on Whole Grains and Fiber-Rich Foods

Fiber is a crucial component of an IC-friendly diet, as it aids in digestion and helps reduce bloating, which can put pressure on the bladder. Whole grains are an excellent source of fiber and provide sustained energy without triggering irritation.

- **Brown Rice, Quinoa, and Oats:** These grains are gentle on the bladder, packed with fiber, and support digestive health. Choose whole grain options over refined grains, as they retain more nutrients and provide more consistent energy.

- **Legumes:** Beans, lentils, and peas are good plant-based sources of protein and fiber. They support overall gut health, though be mindful if legumes cause gas or bloating, which can aggravate symptoms in some individuals.

6. Stock Up on Anti-Inflammatory Ingredients

Since IC is associated with bladder inflammation, incorporating anti-inflammatory foods into your diet can play a vital role in managing symptoms. Look for ingredients that naturally reduce inflammation and help soothe the bladder.

- **Turmeric:** Ground turmeric or fresh turmeric root can be added to soups, stews, teas, or even smoothies. Curcumin, the active compound in turmeric, is known for its anti-inflammatory properties.

- **Ginger:** Fresh or ground ginger is another powerful anti-inflammatory ingredient. Add it to smoothies, stir-fries, or make soothing ginger tea to reduce irritation.

7. Plan for Meal Prep and Storage

Having a well-stocked kitchen with bladder-friendly foods ensures that you always have the right ingredients on hand when it's time to prepare meals. Meal prepping can be a helpful strategy for those with busy schedules, as it allows you to create meals in advance that are both soothing and nourishing.

- **Pre-Chop Vegetables:** Pre-chop vegetables like zucchini, carrots, or bell peppers and store them in the fridge for easy access when preparing meals.

- **Batch Cook Grains:** Cook large batches of brown rice, quinoa, or oats to use as the base for meals throughout the week. These grains store well in the fridge and can be easily reheated.

Following these shopping tips will let you ensure that your kitchen is stocked with foods that support your bladder health, making it easier to stick to a diet that helps manage IC. With careful label reading, smart substitutions, and a focus on whole, fresh ingredients, you'll be able to create a nourishing and soothing diet that helps keep IC symptoms in check.

Chapter 3: IC-Friendly Recipes

BREAKFAST RECIPES

1. Oatmeal with Banana and Almond Butter

Prep Time: 5 minutes
Cook Time: 5 minutes
Total Time: 10 minutes
Servings: 1
Yield: 1 serving

Ingredients:

- 1/2 cup oats
- 1 tablespoon almond butter
- 1 ripe banana, sliced
- 1 teaspoon honey (optional)

How to Prepare:

1. In a small pot, add the oats and enough water or unsweetened almond milk to cover them.
2. Bring to a boil, then reduce to a simmer. Stir occasionally until the oats are soft and the mixture thickens, about 5 minutes.
3. Once the oats are cooked, transfer them to a bowl.
4. Top with sliced banana, almond butter, and a drizzle of honey, if desired.
5. Serve warm and enjoy your soothing breakfast.

Nutrition Facts (per serving):

- Calories: 300
- Protein: 6g
- Fat: 12g
- Carbs: 42g

2. Coconut Yogurt Parfait with Melon and Blueberries

Prep Time: 5 minutes
Cook Time: 0 minutes
Total Time: 5 minutes
Servings: 1
Yield: 1 serving

Ingredients:
- 1/2 cup unsweetened coconut yogurt
- 1/2 cup honeydew melon, diced
- 1/4 cup blueberries
- 1 tablespoon chia seeds

How to Prepare:
1. In a bowl, layer the coconut yogurt, diced honeydew melon, and blueberries.
2. Sprinkle the chia seeds on top for an added boost of fiber.
3. Serve immediately for a refreshing and easy breakfast.

Nutrition Facts (per serving):
- Calories: 200
- Protein: 4g
- Fat: 10g
- Carbs: 25g

3. Scrambled Eggs with Spinach and Zucchini

Prep Time: 5 minutes
Cook Time: 5 minutes
Total Time: 10 minutes
Servings: 1
Yield: 1 serving

Ingredients:

- 2 eggs
- 1/4 cup spinach, chopped
- 1/4 zucchini, diced
- 1 teaspoon olive oil
- Salt (optional)

How to Prepare:

1. Heat olive oil in a skillet over medium heat.
2. Add diced zucchini and cook for 2-3 minutes until slightly tender.
3. Add chopped spinach and cook for another minute.
4. In a bowl, whisk the eggs, then pour them over the vegetables in the skillet.
5. Stir gently until the eggs are scrambled and cooked through, about 2-3 minutes.
6. Add salt to taste, if desired.
7. Serve warm.

Nutrition Facts (per serving):

- Calories: 220
- Protein: 14g
- Fat: 18g
- Carbs: 5g

4. Chia Seed Pudding with Pear and Coconut Flakes

Prep Time: 5 minutes
Cook Time: 0 minutes
Total Time: 5 minutes (plus overnight refrigeration)
Servings: 1
Yield: 1 serving

Ingredients:
- 2 tablespoons chia seeds
- 1/2 cup unsweetened coconut milk
- 1/2 pear, sliced
- 1 tablespoon unsweetened coconut flakes

How to Prepare:
1. In a jar or small bowl, combine the chia seeds and coconut milk.
2. Stir well and refrigerate overnight.
3. In the morning, top with sliced pear and coconut flakes.
4. Serve chilled.

Nutrition Facts (per serving):
- Calories: 180
- Protein: 4g
- Fat: 10g
- Carbs: 25g

5. Rice Pudding with Cinnamon and Pears

Prep Time: 5 minutes
Cook Time: 15 minutes
Total Time: 20 minutes
Servings: 1
Yield: 1 serving

Ingredients:
- 1/2 cup cooked rice
- 1/2 cup unsweetened coconut milk
- 1/2 teaspoon cinnamon
- 1 pear, chopped
- 1 teaspoon honey (optional)

How to Prepare:
1. In a small pot, combine cooked rice and coconut milk.
2. Heat over medium heat, stirring frequently until the mixture becomes creamy, about 10 minutes.
3. Add cinnamon and mix well.
4. Top with chopped pear and a drizzle of honey, if desired.
5. Serve warm.

Nutrition Facts (per serving):
- Calories: 230
- Protein: 4g
- Fat: 9g
- Carbs: 34g

6. Sweet Potato Hash with Turkey Sausage

Prep Time: 5 minutes
Cook Time: 10 minutes
Total Time: 15 minutes
Servings: 1
Yield: 1 serving

Ingredients:

- 1/2 sweet potato, diced
- 2 oz ground turkey (plain)
- 1 teaspoon olive oil
- 1/4 cup spinach, chopped
- Salt (optional)

How to Prepare:

1. Heat olive oil in a skillet over medium heat.
2. Add diced sweet potatoes and cook until tender, about 8 minutes.
3. Add ground turkey and cook until browned, breaking it apart with a spatula, about 5 minutes.
4. Stir in chopped spinach and cook for another 2 minutes.
5. Add salt to taste.
6. Serve warm.

Nutrition Facts (per serving):

- Calories: 300
- Protein: 20g
- Fat: 16g
- Carbs: 30g

7. Quinoa and Blueberry Breakfast Bowl

Prep Time: 5 minutes
Cook Time: 10 minutes
Total Time: 15 minutes
Servings: 1
Yield: 1 serving

Ingredients:
- 1/2 cup cooked quinoa
- 1/4 cup blueberries
- 1/2 cup unsweetened coconut milk
- 1 teaspoon honey (optional)
- 1/4 teaspoon cinnamon

How to Prepare:
1. In a small bowl, combine cooked quinoa and coconut milk.
2. Microwave for 1-2 minutes until warmed through.
3. Top with blueberries, honey (if using), and cinnamon.
4. Serve warm.

Nutrition Facts (per serving):
- Calories: 230
- Protein: 6g
- Fat: 8g
- Carbs: 34g

8. Coconut Flour Pancakes with Maple Syrup

Prep Time: 5 minutes
Cook Time: 10 minutes
Total Time: 15 minutes
Servings: 2
Yield: 2 pancakes

Ingredients:
- 1/2 cup coconut flour
- 2 eggs
- 1/4 cup unsweetened coconut milk
- 1 teaspoon vanilla extract
- 2 teaspoons maple syrup

How to Prepare:
1. In a bowl, whisk together coconut flour, eggs, coconut milk, and vanilla extract until smooth.
2. Heat a non-stick skillet over medium heat and lightly grease with a little coconut oil.
3. Pour the batter into the skillet to form two pancakes. Cook for 2-3 minutes on each side until golden brown.
4. Drizzle with maple syrup.
5. Serve warm.

Nutrition Facts (per serving):
- Calories: 180
- Protein: 8g
- Fat: 14g
- Carbs: 8g

9. Avocado Toast with Hemp Seeds

Prep Time: 5 minutes
Cook Time: 0 minutes
Total Time: 5 minutes
Servings: 1
Yield: 1 serving

Ingredients:

- 1 slice whole grain or gluten-free bread
- 1/2 avocado, mashed
- 1 tablespoon hemp seeds
- 1 teaspoon olive oil

How to Prepare:

1. Toast the slice of bread until golden brown.
2. Spread mashed avocado on top of the toasted bread.
3. Sprinkle with hemp seeds and drizzle with olive oil.
4. Serve immediately.

Nutrition Facts (per serving):

- Calories: 270
- Protein: 8g
- Fat: 20g
- Carbs: 24g

10. Apple Cinnamon Smoothie

Prep Time: 5 minutes
Cook Time: 0 minutes
Total Time: 5 minutes
Servings: 1
Yield: 1 serving

Ingredients:
- 1 apple, cored and chopped
- 1/2 banana
- 1/2 cup unsweetened almond milk
- 1/2 teaspoon cinnamon
- 1 tablespoon flaxseeds

How to Prepare:
1. Add the apple, banana, almond milk, cinnamon, and flaxseeds to a blender.
2. Blend until smooth.
3. Serve immediately in a glass.

Nutrition Facts (per serving):
- Calories: 220
- Protein: 3g
- Fat: 8g
- Carbs: 35g

11. Rice Cake with Almond Butter and Strawberries

Prep Time: 5 minutes
Cook Time: 0 minutes
Total Time: 5 minutes
Servings: 1
Yield: 1 serving

Ingredients:
- 1 plain rice cake
- 1 tablespoon almond butter
- 1/4 cup strawberries, sliced
- 1 teaspoon honey (optional)

How to Prepare:
1. Spread almond butter on top of the rice cake.
2. Top with sliced strawberries.
3. Drizzle with honey, if desired.
4. Serve immediately.

Nutrition Facts (per serving):
- Calories: 180
- Protein: 4g
- Fat: 12g
- Carbs: 18g

12. Vegetable Omelet with Zucchini and Carrot

Prep Time: 5 minutes
Cook Time: 5 minutes
Total Time: 10 minutes
Servings: 1
Yield: 1 serving

Ingredients:
- 2 eggs
- 1/4 cup zucchini, diced
- 1/4 cup carrot, shredded (or finely diced)
- 1/4 cup spinach, chopped
- 1 teaspoon olive oil

How to Prepare:
1. Heat olive oil in a skillet over medium heat.
2. Add the diced zucchini and shredded carrots to the skillet. Sauté for 3-4 minutes until the vegetables soften.
3. In a bowl, whisk the eggs and pour them over the sautéed vegetables in the skillet.
4. Add the chopped spinach to the skillet, stirring lightly to distribute.
5. Cook until the eggs are fully set, about 3-4 minutes, and the vegetables are tender.
6. Serve the omelet warm.

Nutrition Facts (per serving):
- Calories: 220
- Protein: 14g
- Fat: 18g
- Carbs: 6g

13. Non-Dairy Banana Smoothie

Prep Time: 5 minutes
Cook Time: 0 minutes
Total Time: 5 minutes
Servings: 1
Yield: 1 serving

Ingredients:

- 1 banana
- 1/2 cup unsweetened almond milk
- 2 tablespoons flaxseed
- 1/4 cup unsweetened coconut yogurt
- 1 teaspoon honey (optional)

How to Prepare:

1. Add banana, almond milk, flaxseed, coconut yogurt, and honey (if using) to a blender.
2. Blend until smooth.
3. Serve immediately in a glass.

Nutrition Facts (per serving):

- Calories: 250
- Protein: 5g
- Fat: 12g
- Carbs: 32g

14. Baked Oats with Blueberries and Cinnamon

Prep Time: 5 minutes

Cook Time: 25 minutes

Total Time: 30 minutes

Servings: 1

Yield: 1 serving

Ingredients:

- 1/2 cup oats
- 1/4 cup blueberries
- 1/2 cup unsweetened almond milk
- 1/2 teaspoon cinnamon
- 1 teaspoon honey (optional)

How to Prepare:

1. Preheat the oven to 350°F (175°C).
2. In a small oven-safe dish, combine oats, almond milk, cinnamon, and honey.
3. Top with blueberries.
4. Bake for 20-25 minutes, or until oats are tender and liquid is absorbed.
5. Serve warm.

Nutrition Facts (per serving):

- Calories: 220
- Protein: 5g
- Fat: 6g
- Carbs: 38g

15. Coconut Chia Pudding with Kiwi

Prep Time: 5 minutes
Cook Time: 0 minutes
Total Time: 5 minutes (plus overnight refrigeration)
Servings: 1
Yield: 1 serving

Ingredients:
- 2 tablespoons chia seeds
- 1/2 cup unsweetened coconut milk
- 1 kiwi, peeled and sliced
- 1 teaspoon honey (optional)

How to Prepare:
1. In a jar or bowl, mix chia seeds and coconut milk.
2. Stir well and refrigerate overnight.
3. In the morning, top with sliced kiwi and drizzle with honey, if desired.
4. Serve chilled.

Nutrition Facts (per serving):
- Calories: 180
- Protein: 4g
- Fat: 10g
- Carbs: 24g

16. Zucchini Noodles with Avocado Pesto

Prep Time: 10 minutes
Cook Time: 5 minutes
Total Time: 15 minutes
Servings: 1
Yield: 1 serving

Ingredients:

- 1 zucchini, spiralized into noodles
- 1/2 avocado
- 1 tablespoon basil, chopped
- 1 teaspoon olive oil
- Salt (optional)

How to Prepare:

1. Heat olive oil in a skillet over medium heat.
2. Add zucchini noodles and cook for 2-3 minutes until slightly tender.
3. In a blender or food processor, blend avocado, basil, and olive oil until smooth.
4. Toss the zucchini noodles with avocado pesto and serve immediately.

Nutrition Facts (per serving):

- Calories: 210
- Protein: 5g
- Fat: 18g
- Carbs: 14g

17. Oatmeal with Pear and Cinnamon

Prep Time: 5 minutes
Cook Time: 5 minutes
Total Time: 10 minutes
Servings: 1
Yield: 1 serving

Ingredients:
- 1/2 cup oats
- 1 pear, sliced
- 1/2 teaspoon cinnamon
- 1 teaspoon honey (optional)

How to Prepare:
1. In a pot, bring water or almond milk to a boil. Add the oats and simmer for 5 minutes until thick.
2. Add cinnamon and stir.
3. Top with sliced pear and drizzle with honey, if desired.
4. Serve warm.

Nutrition Facts (per serving):
- Calories: 250
- Protein: 6g
- Fat: 8g
- Carbs: 42g

18. Pineapple Coconut Smoothie

Prep Time: 5 minutes
Cook Time: 0 minutes
Total Time: 5 minutes
Servings: 1
Yield: 1 serving

Ingredients:
- 1/2 cup pineapple
- 1/2 cup unsweetened coconut milk
- 1 tablespoon chia seeds
- 1 teaspoon honey (optional)

How to Prepare:
1. Add pineapple, coconut milk, chia seeds, and honey to a blender.
2. Blend until smooth.
3. Serve immediately in a glass.

Nutrition Facts (per serving):
- Calories: 220
- Protein: 4g
- Fat: 10g
- Carbs: 34g

19. Buckwheat Pancakes with Maple Syrup

Prep Time: 5 minutes
Cook Time: 10 minutes
Total Time: 15 minutes
Servings: 2
Yield: 2 pancakes

Ingredients:
- 1/2 cup buckwheat flour
- 2 eggs
- 1/4 cup unsweetened almond milk
- 1 teaspoon vanilla extract
- 2 teaspoons maple syrup

How to Prepare:
1. In a bowl, mix buckwheat flour, eggs, almond milk, and vanilla extract.
2. Heat a non-stick skillet over medium heat and lightly grease with coconut oil.
3. Pour the batter to form pancakes. Cook for 2-3 minutes on each side until golden.
4. Drizzle with maple syrup.
5. Serve warm.

Nutrition Facts (per serving):
- Calories: 200
- Protein: 8g
- Fat: 10g
- Carbs: 22g

20. Coconut and Blueberry Muffins

Prep Time: 10 minutes
Cook Time: 25 minutes
Total Time: 35 minutes
Servings: 6
Yield: 6 muffins

Ingredients:
- 1 cup coconut flour
- 2 eggs
- 1/4 cup unsweetened coconut oil
- 1/4 cup blueberries
- 1 teaspoon honey (optional)

How to Prepare:
1. Preheat the oven to 350°F (175°C).
2. In a bowl, mix coconut flour, eggs, coconut oil, and honey.
3. Fold in the blueberries.
4. Pour batter into muffin tin and bake for 20-25 minutes.
5. Serve warm.

Nutrition Facts (per serving):
- Calories: 220
- Protein: 6g
- Fat: 14g
- Carbs: 18g

LUNCH RECIPES

21. Chicken Salad with Mixed Greens

Prep Time: 15 minutes
Cook Time: 20 minutes
Total Time: 35 minutes
Servings: 2
Yield: 2 servings

Ingredients:

- 1 chicken breast (cooked and shredded)
- 2 cups mixed greens (spinach, lettuce)
- 1 cucumber (sliced)
- 1 tablespoon fresh basil (chopped)
- 1 tablespoon fresh parsley (chopped)
- 1 tablespoon olive oil
- 1 tablespoon lemon juice

How to Prepare:

1. Cook the chicken breast (grill, bake, or boil until fully cooked) and shred it into small pieces.
2. In a large bowl, combine the mixed greens, cucumber slices, basil, and parsley.
3. Add the shredded chicken to the bowl.
4. In a small bowl, whisk together olive oil and lemon juice. Pour over the salad.
5. Toss everything together gently to combine.
6. Serve immediately.

Nutrition Facts (per serving):

- Calories: 280
- Protein: 30g
- Fat: 18g
- Carbs: 5g

22. Quinoa Bowl with Roasted Veggies

Prep Time: 10 minutes
Cook Time: 25 minutes
Total Time: 35 minutes
Servings: 2
Yield: 2 servings

Ingredients:
- 1 cup quinoa (cooked)
- 1 zucchini (chopped)
- 1 sweet potato (peeled and cubed)
- 1 tablespoon olive oil
- 2 cups spinach
- 1 teaspoon fresh basil (chopped)
- Salt to taste

How to Prepare:
1. Preheat your oven to 400°F (200°C).
2. Toss the zucchini and sweet potato with olive oil and salt, then roast on a baking sheet for 20 minutes.
3. While veggies roast, cook quinoa according to package instructions.
4. Once the quinoa is cooked, fluff it with a fork and transfer it to a bowl.
5. Add the roasted veggies, spinach, and basil to the quinoa.
6. Toss everything together and serve warm.

Nutrition Facts (per serving):
- Calories: 350
- Protein: 9g
- Fat: 12g
- Carbs: 50g

23. Rice and Chicken Stir-Fry

Prep Time: 10 minutes
Cook Time: 15 minutes
Total Time: 25 minutes
Servings: 2
Yield: 2 servings

Ingredients:
- 1 cup cooked rice (brown or white)
- 1 chicken breast (cubed)
- 1 zucchini (sliced)
- 2 cups spinach
- 1 tablespoon olive oil
- Mild seasoning (like salt, pepper, and garlic powder)

How to Prepare:
1. Heat olive oil in a large pan over medium heat.
2. Add the cubed chicken and cook until browned and fully cooked (about 7-10 minutes).
3. Add the zucchini and spinach to the pan, and stir-fry for 5-7 minutes until vegetables are tender.
4. Stir in the cooked rice and season with mild spices like salt and garlic powder.
5. Cook for an additional 3-4 minutes until the rice is heated through.
6. Serve warm.

Nutrition Facts (per serving):
- Calories: 400
- Protein: 35g
- Fat: 15g
- Carbs: 35g

24. Turkey and Avocado Lettuce Wraps

Prep Time: 10 minutes
Cook Time: 5 minutes
Total Time: 15 minutes
Servings: 2
Yield: 2 servings

Ingredients:

- 1/2 pound ground turkey (plain)
- 1 avocado (sliced)
- 4 large lettuce leaves (such as Romaine or Butterhead)
- 1 cucumber (sliced)
- 1 tablespoon olive oil

How to Prepare:

1. In a skillet, heat the olive oil over medium heat.
2. Add ground turkey and cook until browned, breaking it apart as it cooks.
3. While turkey cooks, wash and dry the lettuce leaves.
4. Once the turkey is cooked, spoon a portion into each lettuce leaf.
5. Top with sliced avocado and cucumber.
6. Serve as wraps.

Nutrition Facts (per serving):

- Calories: 320
- Protein: 30g
- Fat: 22g
- Carbs: 10g

25. Grilled Salmon with Steamed Asparagus

Prep Time: 10 minutes
Cook Time: 15 minutes
Total Time: 25 minutes
Servings: 2
Yield: 2 servings

Ingredients:
- 2 salmon fillets
- 1 bunch asparagus (trimmed)
- 1 tablespoon olive oil
- 1 tablespoon cucumber juice or pear juice
- Fresh dill (optional)

How to Prepare:
1. Preheat the grill or stovetop grill pan to medium heat.
2. Brush the salmon fillets with olive oil and season with a pinch of salt and cucumber juice or pear juice.
3. Grill the salmon for 4-6 minutes per side, or until cooked through.
4. Meanwhile, steam the asparagus until tender, about 5-7 minutes.
5. Serve the grilled salmon with steamed asparagus and garnish with fresh dill (optional).

Nutrition Facts (per serving):
- Calories: 400
- Protein: 35g
- Fat: 25g
- Carbs: 6g

26. Zucchini Noodles with Chicken and Olive Oil

Prep Time: 10 minutes
Cook Time: 10 minutes
Total Time: 20 minutes
Servings: 2
Yield: 2 servings

Ingredients:
- 2 zucchini (spiralized into noodles)
- 1 chicken breast (sliced)
- 1 tablespoon olive oil
- 1 cup spinach
- 1 tablespoon fresh basil (chopped)

How to Prepare:
1. Heat olive oil in a large skillet over medium heat.
2. Add the chicken slices and cook until browned and cooked through.
3. Add the zucchini noodles and spinach, and cook for an additional 3-5 minutes, until the noodles are tender.
4. Stir in fresh basil.
5. Serve immediately.

Nutrition Facts (per serving):
- Calories: 350
- Protein: 30g
- Fat: 18g
- Carbs: 12g

27. Sweet Potato and Black Bean Bowl

Prep Time: 10 minutes
Cook Time: 25 minutes
Total Time: 35 minutes
Servings: 2
Yield: 2 servings

Ingredients:

- 1 medium sweet potato (peeled and cubed)
- 1 cup black beans (cooked or canned, drained)
- 2 cups spinach
- 1 tablespoon olive oil
- Salt to taste
- Pepper (optional)

How to Prepare:

1. Preheat your oven to 400°F (200°C).
2. Toss the sweet potato cubes with olive oil and a pinch of salt, then spread them out on a baking sheet.
3. Roast for 20-25 minutes, flipping halfway through, until the sweet potato is tender.
4. In a separate pan, sauté spinach in a little olive oil until wilted.
5. In a bowl, combine the roasted sweet potatoes, black beans, and sautéed spinach.
6. Season with salt and pepper to taste and serve warm.

Nutrition Facts (per serving):

- Calories: 350
- Protein: 12g
- Fat: 14g
- Carbs: 45g

28. Quinoa and Veggie Stuffed Sweet Potatoes

Prep Time: 15 minutes
Cook Time: 25 minutes
Total Time: 40 minutes
Servings: 2
Yield: 2 servings

Ingredients:

- 2 medium sweet potatoes (washed and halved)
- 1 cup quinoa (cooked)
- 1 zucchini (chopped)
- 1 cup spinach (chopped)
- 1 tablespoon olive oil
- Salt to taste

How to Prepare:

1. Preheat your oven to 375°F (190°C).
2. Slice the sweet potatoes in half and scoop out some of the flesh to create a cavity for the filling. (You can save the flesh for another use like mashed sweet potatoes.)
3. Place the sweet potato halves on a baking sheet and bake for 20-25 minutes or until tender.
4. While the sweet potatoes bake, heat olive oil in a skillet over medium heat and sauté zucchini and spinach for 5-7 minutes until tender.
5. In a bowl, mix the cooked quinoa with the sautéed vegetables.
6. Once the sweet potatoes are cooked, stuff them with the quinoa and vegetable mixture.
7. Return the stuffed sweet potatoes to the oven for an additional 5 minutes to heat through and allow the tops to brown slightly.
8. Serve warm.

Nutrition Facts (per serving):

Calories: 300; Protein: 10g; Fat: 14g; Carbs: 35g

29. Grilled Chicken with Brown Rice and Green Beans

Prep Time: 10 minutes
Cook Time: 20 minutes
Total Time: 30 minutes
Servings: 2
Yield: 2 servings

Ingredients:

- 2 chicken breasts
- 1 cup brown rice (cooked)
- 1 cup green beans (trimmed)
- 1 tablespoon olive oil
- 1 tablespoon fresh parsley (chopped)

How to Prepare:

1. Preheat the grill or stovetop grill pan to medium heat.
2. Brush the chicken breasts with olive oil and season with salt and pepper.
3. Grill the chicken for 6-8 minutes per side, or until fully cooked.
4. While the chicken cooks, steam the green beans for 5-7 minutes, or until tender.
5. Serve the grilled chicken on a plate with the brown rice and steamed green beans.
6. Garnish with fresh parsley.

Nutrition Facts (per serving):

- Calories: 400
- Protein: 40g
- Fat: 15g
- Carbs: 30g

30. Vegetable Soup with Rice

Prep Time: 10 minutes
Cook Time: 30 minutes
Total Time: 40 minutes
Servings: 4
Yield: 4 servings

Ingredients:
- 2 carrots (peeled and chopped)
- 1 zucchini (chopped)
- 2 cups spinach
- 1 cup cooked rice
- 3 cups mild vegetable broth
- 1 tablespoon olive oil

How to Prepare:
1. In a large pot, heat olive oil over medium heat and sauté carrots and zucchini for 5-7 minutes.
2. Add the vegetable broth and bring to a simmer.
3. Cook for 20 minutes or until the vegetables are tender.
4. Stir in the cooked rice and spinach and cook for an additional 5 minutes.
5. Serve hot.

Nutrition Facts (per serving):
- Calories: 250
- Protein: 7g
- Fat: 8g
- Carbs: 40g

31. Chicken and Spinach Salad with Olive Oil Dressing

Prep Time: 10 minutes
Cook Time: 10 minutes
Total Time: 20 minutes
Servings: 2
Yield: 2 servings

Ingredients:
- 2 chicken breasts (grilled or baked)
- 4 cups spinach
- 1 tablespoon olive oil
- 1 tablespoon lemon juice
- 1 cucumber (sliced)

How to Prepare:
1. Grill or bake the chicken breasts until fully cooked, then slice them thinly.
2. In a large bowl, combine spinach and cucumber.
3. Add the sliced chicken on top.
4. In a small bowl, whisk together olive oil and lemon juice.
5. Drizzle the dressing over the salad and toss gently.
6. Serve immediately.

Nutrition Facts (per serving):
- Calories: 350
- Protein: 40g
- Fat: 18g
- Carbs: 10g

32. Lentil Salad with Cucumber and Tomatoes

Prep Time: 15 minutes
Cook Time: 25 minutes
Total Time: 40 minutes
Servings: 2
Yield: 2 servings

Ingredients:

- 1 cup cooked lentils
- 1 cucumber (sliced)
- 2 medium tomatoes (bland variety)
- 1 tablespoon olive oil
- 1 tablespoon fresh parsley (chopped)

How to Prepare:

1. In a large bowl, combine the cooked lentils, cucumber, and tomatoes.
2. Drizzle with olive oil and toss gently.
3. Garnish with fresh parsley and serve.

Nutrition Facts (per serving):

- Calories: 300
- Protein: 15g
- Fat: 10g
- Carbs: 35g

33. Chicken and Sweet Potato Stew

Prep Time: 10 minutes
Cook Time: 30 minutes
Total Time: 40 minutes
Servings: 4
Yield: 4 servings

Ingredients:
- 2 chicken breasts (cubed)
- 2 medium sweet potatoes (peeled and cubed)
- 2 cups spinach
- 1 tablespoon olive oil
- Mild seasoning (such as salt, pepper, and thyme)

How to Prepare:
1. In a large pot, heat olive oil over medium heat and cook the chicken cubes until browned.
2. Add the sweet potatoes and cook for an additional 5 minutes.
3. Add enough water to cover the ingredients, then bring to a simmer.
4. Cook for 20 minutes, or until the sweet potatoes are tender.
5. Stir in the spinach and cook for an additional 5 minutes.
6. Serve hot.

Nutrition Facts (per serving):
- Calories: 350
- Protein: 30g
- Fat: 15g
- Carbs: 30g

34. Rice and Veggie Casserole

Prep Time: 15 minutes
Cook Time: 35 minutes
Total Time: 50 minutes
Servings: 4
Yield: 4 servings

Ingredients:

- 1 cup cooked rice
- 1 zucchini (chopped)
- 1 cup sweet potatoes (cubed)
- 1 cup spinach (chopped)
- 1 tablespoon olive oil
- Salt to taste

How to Prepare:

1. Preheat your oven to 375°F (190°C).
2. In a large skillet, sauté the zucchini and sweet potatoes in olive oil over medium heat for 7-10 minutes until softened.
3. Add the chopped spinach and cook for another 2-3 minutes until wilted.
4. In a casserole dish, combine the cooked rice and sautéed vegetables.
5. Season with salt and mix well.
6. Cover and bake for 30 minutes.
7. Remove the cover and bake for an additional 5 minutes for a golden top.
8. Serve warm.

Nutrition Facts (per serving):

- Calories: 280
- Protein: 6g
- Fat: 8g
- Carbs: 45g

35. Cucumber and Avocado Sushi Rolls

Prep Time: 15 minutes
Cook Time: 10 minutes
Total Time: 25 minutes
Servings: 2
Yield: 2 servings

Ingredients:
- 1 cucumber (julienned)
- 1 avocado (sliced)
- 1 cup rice (cooked and seasoned)
- 2 sheets nori (seaweed)
- 1 tablespoon olive oil

How to Prepare:
1. Cook the rice and allow it to cool slightly.
2. Lay a sheet of nori on a sushi mat or clean surface.
3. Spread a thin layer of cooked rice onto the nori, leaving a small border at the top.
4. Arrange the cucumber and avocado slices in the center of the rice.
5. Roll the sushi tightly using the mat, pressing gently to seal the edge.
6. Slice the roll into bite-sized pieces and serve.

Nutrition Facts (per serving):
- Calories: 250
- Protein: 6g
- Fat: 15g
- Carbs: 30g

36. Turkey and Cucumber Salad

Prep Time: 10 minutes
Cook Time: 5 minutes
Total Time: 15 minutes
Servings: 2
Yield: 2 servings

Ingredients:

- 1 cup ground turkey (plain, cooked)
- 1 cucumber (sliced)
- 2 cups spinach (chopped)
- 1 tablespoon olive oil
- 1 tablespoon cucumber juice

How to Prepare:

1. In a skillet, cook the ground turkey over medium heat until browned and cooked through.
2. In a large bowl, combine the cooked turkey, sliced cucumber, and spinach.
3. Drizzle with olive oil and cucumber juice.
4. Toss gently and serve immediately.

Nutrition Facts (per serving):

- Calories: 300
- Protein: 35g
- Fat: 15g
- Carbs: 10g

37. Egg Salad with Avocado and Spinach

Prep Time: 10 minutes
Cook Time: 10 minutes
Total Time: 20 minutes
Servings: 2
Yield: 2 servings

Ingredients:

- 4 boiled eggs (peeled and chopped)
- 1 avocado (sliced)
- 1 cup spinach (chopped)
- 1 tablespoon olive oil
- 1 tablespoon pear juice
- Salt to taste

How to Prepare:

1. Boil the eggs and chop them into pieces.
2. In a bowl, combine the chopped eggs, avocado slices, and spinach.
3. Drizzle with olive oil and pear juice.
4. Season with salt and toss gently.
5. Serve chilled or at room temperature.

Nutrition Facts (per serving):

- Calories: 350
- Protein: 20g
- Fat: 25g
- Carbs: 15g

38. Grilled Veggie Wrap with Hummus

Prep Time: 15 minutes
Cook Time: 15 minutes
Total Time: 30 minutes
Servings: 2
Yield: 2 servings

Ingredients:
- 1 zucchini (sliced)
- 1 medium carrot (sliced or julienned)
- 2 cups spinach
- 2 gluten-free tortillas
- 3 tablespoons hummus
- 1 tablespoon olive oil

How to Prepare:
1. Preheat a grill or grill pan over medium heat.
2. Toss the zucchini and carrot slices in olive oil and grill for 5-7 minutes until tender and slightly charred.
3. Lay the grilled vegetables on a tortilla, adding spinach and a tablespoon of hummus.
4. Roll the tortilla into a wrap and slice it into halves.
5. Serve immediately.

Nutrition Facts (per serving):
- Calories: 300
- Protein: 10g
- Fat: 15g
- Carbs: 35g

39. Baked Chicken with Roasted Carrots and Quinoa

Prep Time: 15 minutes
Cook Time: 35 minutes
Total Time: 50 minutes
Servings: 2
Yield: 2 servings

Ingredients:
- 2 chicken breasts
- 2 carrots (peeled and chopped)
- 1 cup quinoa (cooked)
- 1 tablespoon olive oil
- 1 tablespoon fresh parsley (chopped)

How to Prepare:
1. Preheat your oven to 375°F (190°C).
2. Drizzle olive oil over the chicken breasts and season with salt and pepper.
3. Place the chicken on a baking sheet and arrange the carrots around it.
4. Roast in the oven for 30-35 minutes, or until the chicken is fully cooked and the carrots are tender.
5. Serve with cooked quinoa, garnished with fresh parsley.

Nutrition Facts (per serving):
- Calories: 400
- Protein: 40g
- Fat: 15g
- Carbs: 35g

40. Coconut Milk Chicken Soup

Prep Time: 10 minutes
Cook Time: 25 minutes
Total Time: 35 minutes
Servings: 4
Yield: 4 servings

Ingredients:
- 2 chicken breasts (cubed)
- 2 cups coconut milk (unsweetened)
- 1 cup spinach (chopped)
- 1 zucchini (sliced)
- Mild seasoning (such as salt and thyme)

How to Prepare:
1. In a large pot, cook the cubed chicken in a little olive oil until browned.
2. Add the coconut milk and bring to a simmer.
3. Add the zucchini and cook for 10 minutes until tender.
4. Stir in the spinach and cook for an additional 5 minutes.
5. Season with salt and thyme to taste.
6. Serve hot.

Nutrition Facts (per serving):
- Calories: 350
- Protein: 30g
- Fat: 20g
- Carbs: 10g

DINNER RECIPES

41. Baked Salmon with Sweet Potatoes and Steamed Broccoli

Prep Time: 10 minutes *Cook Time: 30 minutes* *Total Time: 40 minutes*
Servings: 2 *Yield: 2 servings*

Ingredients:

- 2 salmon fillets (approximately 6 oz each)
- 2 medium sweet potatoes, peeled and cut into cubes
- 1 large head of broccoli, cut into florets
- 2 tablespoons olive oil
- 1 tablespoon pear juice
- Fresh dill (optional, for garnish)

How to Prepare:

1. Preheat the oven to 400°F (200°C).
2. Place the salmon fillets on a baking sheet and drizzle with 1 tablespoon of olive oil. Season with a pinch of salt and pepper (optional). Drizzle pear juice over the salmon fillets.
3. Arrange the sweet potato cubes on another baking sheet and drizzle with the remaining tablespoon of olive oil. Roast in the oven for 25-30 minutes, or until tender, flipping halfway through.
4. While the salmon and sweet potatoes are baking, steam the broccoli florets for 5-7 minutes, or until tender but still vibrant.
5. Once everything is cooked, serve the salmon with roasted sweet potatoes and steamed broccoli. Garnish with fresh dill if desired.

Nutrition Facts (per serving):

- Calories: 450
- Protein: 35g
- Fat: 22g

- Carbs: 35g

42. Turkey Meatballs with Brown Rice and Squash

Prep Time: 15 minutes *Cook Time: 25 minutes* *Total Time: 40 minutes*
Servings: 4 *Yield: 4 servings*

Ingredients:

- 1 lb ground turkey (plain)
- 1 cup brown rice
- 1 medium zucchini, diced
- 1 medium yellow squash, diced
- 2 tablespoons olive oil
- 1 teaspoon garlic powder
- 1 teaspoon dried basil
- Salt (optional)

How to Prepare:

1. Preheat the oven to 375°F (190°C).
2. In a bowl, mix the ground turkey, garlic powder, dried basil, and salt (optional) until fully combined. Form the mixture into meatballs (about 1 inch in diameter) and place them on a baking sheet.
3. Bake the meatballs for 15-20 minutes or until fully cooked (internal temperature should reach 165°F or 75°C).
4. While the meatballs are baking, cook the brown rice according to the package instructions.
5. In a large pan, heat olive oil over medium heat. Add the diced zucchini and squash, and sauté for 5-7 minutes, until tender.
6. Serve the turkey meatballs with brown rice and sautéed zucchini and squash.

Nutrition Facts (per serving):

- Calories: 370
- Protein: 32g
- Fat: 18g
- Carbs: 28g

43. Vegetable Soup with Carrots, Zucchini, and Celery

Prep Time: 10 minutes
Cook Time: 25 minutes
Total Time: 35 minutes
Servings: 4
Yield: 4 servings

Ingredients:

- 3 large carrots, peeled and sliced
- 2 medium zucchinis, sliced
- 3 stalks celery, chopped
- 4 cups vegetable broth (low-sodium, mild)
- 1 tablespoon olive oil
- Salt (optional)

How to Prepare:

1. Heat olive oil in a large pot over medium heat.
2. Add the carrots, zucchini, and celery. Sauté for 5 minutes until the vegetables begin to soften.
3. Add the vegetable broth to the pot and bring to a simmer.
4. Let the soup simmer for 20 minutes, or until the vegetables are tender.
5. Season with salt (optional) to taste. Serve warm.

Nutrition Facts (per serving):

- Calories: 150
- Protein: 4g
- Fat: 7g
- Carbs: 20g

44. Chicken and Quinoa Stir Fry with Spinach

Prep Time: 10 minutes
Cook Time: 15 minutes
Total Time: 25 minutes
Servings: 4
Yield: 4 servings

Ingredients:
- 2 chicken breasts, diced
- 1 cup quinoa (rinsed)
- 2 cups fresh spinach
- 1 medium zucchini or 1 carrot, diced
- 2 tablespoons olive oil
- Salt (optional)
- 1 tablespoon mild seasoning (such as dried basil or oregano)

How to Prepare:
1. Cook the quinoa according to the package instructions. Set aside.
2. Heat olive oil in a large pan over medium heat. Add the diced chicken and sauté for 6-8 minutes until fully cooked.
3. Add the diced zucchini (or carrot) and spinach to the pan, and cook for 2-3 minutes until the spinach wilts and the zucchini/carrot is tender.
4. Stir in the cooked quinoa and seasoning, then cook for an additional 2-3 minutes, ensuring everything is evenly mixed.
5. Season with salt (optional), then serve.

Nutrition Facts (per serving):
- Calories: 400
- Protein: 35g
- Fat: 16g
- Carbs: 30g

45. Grilled Chicken with Roasted Vegetables

Prep Time: 10 minutes
Cook Time: 30 minutes
Total Time: 40 minutes
Servings: 4
Yield: 4 servings

Ingredients:
- 4 chicken breasts
- 2 medium carrots, peeled and cut into sticks
- 2 medium zucchinis, sliced
- 2 tablespoons olive oil
- 1 teaspoon rosemary
- Salt (optional)

How to Prepare:
1. Preheat the oven to 400°F (200°C).
2. Toss the carrots and zucchini with olive oil, rosemary, and salt (optional). Spread them in a single layer on a baking sheet.
3. Grill the chicken breasts over medium heat for 6-8 minutes per side, or until the internal temperature reaches 165°F (75°C).
4. Roast the vegetables in the oven for 25-30 minutes, turning halfway through, until tender and golden.
5. Serve the grilled chicken with the roasted vegetables.

Nutrition Facts (per serving):
- Calories: 375
- Protein: 40g
- Fat: 18g
- Carbs: 22g

46. Baked Cod with Steamed Carrots and Sweet Potatoes

Prep Time: 10 minutes
Cook Time: 30 minutes
Total Time: 40 minutes
Servings: 4
Yield: 4 servings

Ingredients:
- 4 cod fillets (approximately 6 oz each)
- 2 medium carrots, peeled and cut into sticks
- 2 medium sweet potatoes, peeled and cut into cubes
- 2 tablespoons olive oil
- 1 tablespoon parsley
- 1 tablespoon pear juice

How to Prepare:
1. Preheat the oven to 375°F (190°C).
2. Place the cod fillets on a baking sheet. Drizzle with 1 tablespoon of olive oil, season with salt (optional), and top with pear juice.
3. Arrange the sweet potato cubes on a separate baking sheet, drizzle with the remaining tablespoon of olive oil, and roast for 25-30 minutes, or until tender.
4. Steam the carrots for 5-7 minutes, or until tender.
5. Serve the baked cod with roasted sweet potatoes and steamed carrots, garnished with parsley.

Nutrition Facts (per serving):
- Calories: 380
- Protein: 32g
- Fat: 15g
- Carbs: 35g

47. Chicken and Sweet Potato Stew

Prep Time: 10 minutes

Cook Time: 35 minutes

Total Time: 45 minutes

Servings: 4

Yield: 4 servings

Ingredients:
- 2 chicken breasts, diced
- 2 medium sweet potatoes, peeled and cubed
- 2 medium carrots, peeled and sliced
- 2 tablespoons olive oil
- 2 cups spinach (optional)
- 1 teaspoon mild seasoning (such as thyme or rosemary)
- Salt (optional)

How to Prepare:
1. Heat olive oil in a large pot over medium heat. Add the diced chicken and sauté until browned, about 6-8 minutes.
2. Add the sweet potatoes, carrots, and mild seasoning, and stir to combine.
3. Pour in enough water or low-sodium broth to cover the vegetables and chicken. Bring to a simmer and cook for 25-30 minutes, or until the sweet potatoes and carrots are tender.
4. Stir in the spinach (optional) and cook for an additional 5 minutes.
5. Season with salt (optional), then serve warm.

Nutrition Facts (per serving):
- Calories: 375
- Protein: 35g
- Fat: 15g
- Carbs: 35g

48. Stuffed Yellow Squash with Quinoa and Turkey

Prep Time: 15 minutes   *Cook Time: 30 minutes*   *Total Time: 45 minutes*
Servings: 4   *Yield: 4 servings*

Ingredients:

- 4 medium yellow squash (cut in half lengthwise and hollowed out)
- 1 cup quinoa (rinsed)
- 1 lb ground turkey (plain)
- 1 medium zucchini, diced
- 2 tablespoons olive oil
- 1 tablespoon fresh basil, chopped

How to Prepare:

1. Preheat the oven to 375°F (190°C).
2. Cut the yellow squash in half lengthwise and remove the seeds and pulp to create a hollow center. Place the squash halves in a baking dish.
3. Cook the quinoa according to the package instructions. Set aside.
4. Heat olive oil in a large skillet over medium heat. Add the ground turkey and cook until browned, about 7-8 minutes.
5. Add the diced zucchini to the skillet and cook for an additional 3-4 minutes until softened.
6. Stir in the cooked quinoa and fresh basil.
7. Stuff each yellow squash half with the turkey and quinoa mixture, and place them in the baking dish.
8. Cover with aluminum foil and bake for 25-30 minutes, or until the squash is tender.
9. Serve warm.

Nutrition Facts (per serving):

- Calories: 350
- Protein: 30g
- Fat: 15g
- Carbs: 30g

49. Herb Grilled Salmon with Brown Rice

Prep Time: 10 minutes
Cook Time: 15 minutes
Total Time: 25 minutes
Servings: 2
Yield: 2 servings

Ingredients:
- 2 salmon fillets (approximately 6 oz each)
- 1 cup brown rice
- 1 tablespoon pear juice
- 1 tablespoon olive oil
- 1 tablespoon fresh dill, chopped

How to Prepare:
1. Cook the brown rice according to the package instructions. Set aside.
2. Preheat the grill to medium-high heat.
3. Drizzle the salmon fillets with olive oil and top with pear juice and fresh dill.
4. Grill the salmon for 5-7 minutes on each side, or until fully cooked and the internal temperature reaches 145°F (63°C).
5. Serve the grilled salmon over brown rice. Garnish with extra fresh dill.

Nutrition Facts (per serving):
- Calories: 400
- Protein: 35g
- Fat: 22g
- Carbs: 30g

50. Vegetable Stir Fry with Tofu and Brown Rice

Prep Time: 10 minutes *Cook Time: 15 minutes* *Total Time: 25 minutes*
Servings: 4 *Yield: 4 servings*

Ingredients:
- 1 block firm tofu, drained and cubed
- 1 cup brown rice
- 1 zucchini, sliced
- 1 bell pepper, sliced
- 1 cup spinach (optional)
- 2 tablespoons olive oil
- 1 tablespoon coconut aminos

How to Prepare:
1. Cook the brown rice according to the package instructions. Set aside.
2. Heat 1 tablespoon of olive oil in a large skillet or wok over medium heat. Add the tofu and cook until golden on all sides, about 8 minutes.
3. Remove the tofu from the skillet and set aside.
4. In the same skillet, heat the remaining olive oil. Add the zucchini and bell pepper, and sauté for 5-7 minutes until softened.
5. Stir in the spinach (optional) and cook for an additional 2 minutes until wilted.
6. Return the tofu to the skillet and drizzle with coconut aminos. Stir to combine and heat through.
7. Serve the stir fry with brown rice.

Nutrition Facts (per serving):
- Calories: 350
- Protein: 18g
- Fat: 18g
- Carbs: 30g

51. Grilled Chicken with Avocado and Cucumber Salad

Prep Time: 10 minutes
Cook Time: 10 minutes
Total Time: 20 minutes
Servings: 2
Yield: 2 servings

Ingredients:

- 2 chicken breasts
- 1 avocado, sliced
- 1 cucumber, sliced
- 1 tablespoon olive oil
- 1 tablespoon pear juice
- 1 tablespoon fresh parsley, chopped

How to Prepare:

1. Preheat the grill to medium-high heat.
2. Grill the chicken breasts for 6-8 minutes per side, or until the internal temperature reaches 165°F (75°C).
3. In a bowl, combine the sliced avocado, cucumber, olive oil, pear juice, and parsley. Toss gently.
4. Serve the grilled chicken with the avocado and cucumber salad.

Nutrition Facts (per serving):

- Calories: 420
- Protein: 40g
- Fat: 25g
- Carbs: 15g

52. Baked Chicken with Steamed Asparagus and Quinoa

Prep Time: 10 minutes
Cook Time: 30 minutes
Total Time: 40 minutes
Servings: 4
Yield: 4 servings

Ingredients:
- 4 chicken breasts
- 2 cups asparagus, trimmed
- 1 cup quinoa (rinsed)
- 2 tablespoons olive oil
- 1 tablespoon coconut water
- Fresh parsley (for garnish)

How to Prepare:
1. Preheat the oven to 375°F (190°C).
2. Drizzle the chicken breasts with olive oil and season with salt (optional). Bake for 25-30 minutes, or until the internal temperature reaches 165°F (75°C).
3. While the chicken is baking, cook the quinoa according to the package instructions.
4. Steam the asparagus for 5-7 minutes until tender.
5. Serve the baked chicken with quinoa and steamed asparagus. Garnish with fresh parsley and a drizzle of coconut water.

Nutrition Facts (per serving):
- Calories: 370
- Protein: 40g
- Fat: 15g
- Carbs: 30g

53. Quinoa and Vegetable Patties

Prep Time: 15 minutes
Cook Time: 15 minutes
Total Time: 30 minutes
Servings: 4
Yield: 4 servings

Ingredients:

- 1 cup quinoa (rinsed)
- 1 medium zucchini, grated
- 1 medium carrot, grated
- 1 egg (optional)
- 2 tablespoons olive oil
- Salt (optional)

How to Prepare:

1. Cook the quinoa according to the package instructions. Let it cool.
2. In a large bowl, combine the cooked quinoa, grated zucchini, grated carrot, and egg (if using). Mix until well combined.
3. Form the mixture into small patties.
4. Heat olive oil in a skillet over medium heat. Cook the patties for 4-5 minutes on each side, or until golden brown.
5. Serve warm as a side or main dish.

Nutrition Facts (per serving):

- Calories: 200
- Protein: 8g
- Fat: 9g
- Carbs: 25g

54. Lentil Soup with Carrots and Zucchini

Prep Time: 10 minutes
Cook Time: 30 minutes
Total Time: 40 minutes
Servings: 4
Yield: 4 servings

Ingredients:
- 1 cup cooked lentils
- 2 medium carrots, peeled and sliced
- 1 medium zucchini, sliced
- 2 cups vegetable broth (low-sodium, mild)
- 2 tablespoons olive oil

How to Prepare:
1. Heat olive oil in a large pot over medium heat. Add the carrots and zucchini, and sauté for 5 minutes.
2. Add the cooked lentils and vegetable broth to the pot. Stir to combine.
3. Bring to a simmer and cook for 20-25 minutes until the vegetables are tender.
4. Season with salt (optional) and serve warm.

Nutrition Facts (per serving):
- Calories: 230
- Protein: 12g
- Fat: 7g
- Carbs: 30g

55. Baked Turkey with Roasted Carrots and Green Beans

Prep Time: 10 minutes
Cook Time: 40 minutes
Total Time: 50 minutes
Servings: 4
Yield: 4 servings

Ingredients:
- 1 lb turkey breast
- 2 medium carrots, peeled and cut into sticks
- 1 cup green beans, trimmed
- 2 tablespoons olive oil
- 1 tablespoon fresh rosemary
- 1 tablespoon fresh parsley

How to Prepare:
1. Preheat the oven to 375°F (190°C).
2. Place the turkey breast in a baking dish and drizzle with olive oil. Season with salt (optional) and sprinkle with rosemary.
3. Arrange the carrots and green beans around the turkey in the baking dish.
4. Roast in the oven for 35-40 minutes or until the turkey reaches an internal temperature of 165°F (75°C).
5. Remove from the oven, garnish with fresh parsley, and serve warm.

Nutrition Facts (per serving):
- Calories: 350
- Protein: 40g
- Fat: 15g
- Carbs: 20g

56. Zucchini Noodles with Grilled Chicken and Olive Oil

Prep Time: 10 minutes
Cook Time: 10 minutes
Total Time: 20 minutes
Servings: 2
Yield: 2 servings

Ingredients:
- 2 medium zucchinis, spiralized into noodles
- 2 chicken breasts
- 2 tablespoons olive oil
- 1 tablespoon fresh basil, chopped
- 1 tablespoon fresh parsley, chopped
- Salt (optional)

How to Prepare:
1. Preheat the grill to medium-high heat.
2. Season the chicken breasts with olive oil and grill for 6-8 minutes per side or until fully cooked.
3. While the chicken is grilling, heat olive oil in a skillet over medium heat. Add the zucchini noodles and sauté for 2-3 minutes until slightly tender.
4. Slice the grilled chicken and place on top of the zucchini noodles.
5. Garnish with fresh basil and parsley, and serve warm.

Nutrition Facts (per serving):
- Calories: 400
- Protein: 35g
- Fat: 20g
- Carbs: 15g

57. Chicken and Avocado Lettuce Wraps

Prep Time: 10 minutes
Cook Time: 10 minutes
Total Time: 20 minutes
Servings: 4
Yield: 4 servings

Ingredients:
- 2 chicken breasts, cooked and shredded
- 1 avocado, sliced
- 1 cucumber, sliced
- 1 head of lettuce (preferably Romaine or Butterhead)
- 1 tablespoon olive oil
- 1 tablespoon pear juice

How to Prepare:
1. Cook the chicken breasts and shred them once fully cooked.
2. Wash and separate the lettuce leaves.
3. Assemble the wraps by placing a few spoonfuls of shredded chicken, slices of avocado, and cucumber on each lettuce leaf.
4. Drizzle with olive oil and pear juice, then roll up the lettuce leaf to create the wrap.
5. Serve immediately as a fresh, light dinner.

Nutrition Facts (per serving):
- Calories: 280
- Protein: 25g
- Fat: 18g
- Carbs: 10g

58. Grilled Veggie Skewers with Brown Rice

Prep Time: 15 minutes

Cook Time: 20 minutes

Total Time: 35 minutes

Servings: 4

Yield: 4 servings

Ingredients:
- 1 zucchini, sliced
- 1 yellow squash, cut into chunks
- 1 cup carrots, cut into rounds or sticks
- 1 cup brown rice
- 2 tablespoons olive oil
- 1 tablespoon rosemary, chopped

How to Prepare:
1. Preheat the grill to medium-high heat.
2. Thread the zucchini, yellow squash, and carrots onto skewers. Drizzle with olive oil and sprinkle with rosemary.
3. Grill the vegetable skewers for 8-10 minutes, turning occasionally, until they are tender and slightly charred.
4. Cook the brown rice according to the package instructions.
5. Serve the grilled vegetable skewers over the brown rice.

Nutrition Facts (per serving):
- Calories: 350
- Protein: 8g
- Fat: 18g
- Carbs: 40g

59. Pork Tenderloin with Roasted Carrots and Spinach

Prep Time: 10 minutes

Cook Time: 35 minutes

Total Time: 45 minutes

Servings: 4

Yield: 4 servings

Ingredients:

- 1 lb pork tenderloin
- 2 medium carrots, peeled and sliced
- 2 cups spinach (optional)
- 2 tablespoons olive oil
- 1 tablespoon garlic, minced
- 1 tablespoon rosemary

How to Prepare:

1. Preheat the oven to 375°F (190°C).
2. Rub the pork tenderloin with olive oil, garlic, and rosemary. Place on a baking sheet.
3. Roast for 25-30 minutes, or until the internal temperature reaches 145°F (63°C).
4. While the pork roasts, steam or sauté the carrots and spinach in a pan with olive oil for 8-10 minutes.
5. Slice the pork tenderloin and serve with roasted carrots and spinach.

Nutrition Facts (per serving):

- Calories: 370
- Protein: 40g
- Fat: 18g
- Carbs: 25g

60. Coconut Milk Chicken Curry with Steamed Vegetables

Prep Time: 10 minutes

Cook Time: 25 minutes

Total Time: 35 minutes

Servings: 4

Yield: 4 servings

Ingredients:

- 2 chicken breasts, diced
- 1 can coconut milk (unsweetened)
- 2 medium carrots, sliced
- 1 zucchini, sliced
- 1 tablespoon mild curry powder
- 2 tablespoons olive oil
- 1 cup spinach (optional)

How to Prepare:

1. Heat olive oil in a large skillet over medium heat. Add the chicken and cook until browned, about 6-8 minutes.
2. Add the curry powder and stir to coat the chicken.
3. Pour in the coconut milk and bring to a simmer. Cook for 10 minutes.
4. Add the carrots, zucchini, and spinach (optional) to the skillet, and cook for an additional 10 minutes, or until the vegetables are tender.
5. Serve warm.

Nutrition Facts (per serving):

- Calories: 400
- Protein: 35g
- Fat: 24g
- Carbs: 25g
-

SNACK RECIPES

61. Homemade Granola Bars

Prep Time: 15 minutes   *Cook Time: 20 minutes*   *Total Time: 35 minutes*
Servings: 12 bars   *Yield: 12 bars*

Ingredients:
- 2 cups oats
- 1/4 cup honey
- 1/2 cup mild fruits (pears or apples), diced
- 1/4 cup unsweetened coconut flakes
- 1 tablespoon chia seeds
- 1/4 cup almond butter

How to Prepare:
1. Preheat the oven to 350°F (175°C).
2. In a large mixing bowl, combine the oats, honey, diced fruits, coconut flakes, chia seeds, and almond butter.
3. Mix well until all ingredients are evenly combined.
4. Press the mixture into a baking dish lined with parchment paper.
5. Bake for 15-20 minutes until golden brown.
6. Let the granola bars cool before cutting into squares.
7. Serve and enjoy!

Nutrition Facts (per serving):
- Calories: 120
- Protein: 3g
- Fat: 6g
- Carbs: 14g

62. Rice Cakes with Avocado

Prep Time: 5 minutes
Cook Time: 0 minutes
Total Time: 5 minutes
Servings: 1
Yield: 1 serving

Ingredients:
- 2 plain rice cakes
- 1/2 avocado
- 1 teaspoon olive oil
- 1 teaspoon hemp seeds

How to Prepare:
1. Spread the olive oil evenly over the rice cakes.
2. Mash the avocado and spread it over the rice cakes.
3. Sprinkle hemp seeds on top.
4. Serve immediately.

Nutrition Facts (per serving):
- Calories: 200
- Protein: 4g
- Fat: 12g
- Carbs: 22g

63. Non-Dairy Yogurt Parfait

Prep Time: 5 minutes
Cook Time: 0 minutes
Total Time: 5 minutes
Servings: 1
Yield: 1 serving

Ingredients:

- 1/2 cup unsweetened almond milk yogurt
- 1/4 cup blueberries
- 2 tablespoons oats
- 1 tablespoon chia seeds

How to Prepare:

1. In a small bowl or glass, layer the yogurt, blueberries, oats, and chia seeds.
2. Repeat the layers as needed.
3. Serve chilled.

Nutrition Facts (per serving):

- Calories: 140
- Protein: 5g
- Fat: 6g
- Carbs: 17g

64. Carrot and Cucumber Sticks with Hummus

Prep Time: 10 minutes
Cook Time: 0 minutes
Total Time: 10 minutes
Servings: 2
Yield: 2 servings

Ingredients:

- 1 carrot, cut into sticks
- 1 cucumber, cut into sticks
- 1/4 cup homemade hummus (olive oil, tahini, garlic)

How to Prepare:

1. Peel and slice the carrot and cucumber into sticks.
2. Serve with homemade hummus for dipping.

Nutrition Facts (per serving):

- Calories: 150
- Protein: 4g
- Fat: 9g
- Carbs: 15g

65. Baked Apple Chips

Prep Time: 10 minutes
Cook Time: 1 hour
Total Time: 1 hour 10 minutes
Servings: 4
Yield: 4 servings

Ingredients:
- 2 apples, thinly sliced
- 1/2 teaspoon cinnamon (optional)

How to Prepare:
1. Preheat the oven to 200°F (95°C).
2. Arrange the apple slices on a baking sheet lined with parchment paper.
3. Sprinkle with cinnamon (optional).
4. Bake for 1 hour, flipping halfway through, until crisp.
5. Serve once cooled.

Nutrition Facts (per serving):
- Calories: 80
- Protein: 0g
- Fat: 0g
- Carbs: 21g

66. Banana and Almond Butter Bites

Prep Time: 5 minutes

Cook Time: 0 minutes

Total Time: 5 minutes

Servings: 1

Yield: 1 serving

Ingredients:

- 1 banana
- 2 tablespoons almond butter

How to Prepare:

1. Slice the banana into rounds.
2. Spread almond butter on top of each slice.
3. Serve immediately.

Nutrition Facts (per serving):

- Calories: 210
- Protein: 5g
- Fat: 16g
- Carbs: 22g

67. Zucchini Chips

Prep Time: 10 minutes
Cook Time: 1 hour
Total Time: 1 hour 10 minutes
Servings: 4
Yield: 4 servings

Ingredients:

- 1 zucchini, sliced thin
- 1 tablespoon olive oil
- 1/4 teaspoon sea salt (optional)

How to Prepare:

1. Preheat the oven to 200°F (95°C).
2. Toss the zucchini slices in olive oil and sea salt.
3. Arrange on a baking sheet lined with parchment paper.
4. Bake for 1 hour, flipping halfway through, until crispy.
5. Serve once cooled.

Nutrition Facts (per serving):

- Calories: 50
- Protein: 1g
- Fat: 4g
- Carbs: 6g

68. Coconut Chia Pudding

Prep Time: 5 minutes
Cook Time: 0 minutes
Total Time: 5 minutes + 2 hours chilling
Servings: 1
Yield: 1 serving

Ingredients:

- 2 tablespoons chia seeds
- 1/2 cup coconut milk (unsweetened)
- 1 teaspoon honey (optional)

How to Prepare:

1. In a bowl, combine chia seeds and coconut milk.
2. Stir well and let sit in the refrigerator for 2 hours or overnight.
3. Stir again before serving and enjoy!

Nutrition Facts (per serving):

- Calories: 150
- Protein: 4g
- Fat: 9g
- Carbs: 14g

69. Rice Cake with Almond Butter and Pear Slices

Prep Time: 5 minutes
Cook Time: 0 minutes
Total Time: 5 minutes
Servings: 1
Yield: 1 serving

Ingredients:

- 1 plain rice cake
- 1 tablespoon almond butter
- 1/2 pear, sliced

How to Prepare:

1. Spread almond butter evenly over the rice cake.
2. Arrange pear slices on top.
3. Serve immediately.

Nutrition Facts (per serving):

- Calories: 160
- Protein: 4g
- Fat: 10g
- Carbs: 18g

70. Apple Slices with Almond Butter

Prep Time: 5 minutes
Cook Time: 0 minutes
Total Time: 5 minutes
Servings: 1
Yield: 1 serving

Ingredients:
- 1 apple, sliced
- 2 tablespoons almond butter

How to Prepare:
1. Slice the apple into wedges.
2. Dip or spread almond butter on each slice.
3. Serve immediately.

Nutrition Facts (per serving):
- Calories: 220
- Protein: 5g
- Fat: 16g
- Carbs: 23g

71. Oatmeal Energy Balls

Prep Time: 10 minutes
Cook Time: 0 minutes
Total Time: 10 minutes
Servings: 12 balls
Yield: 12 balls

Ingredients:

- 1 cup oats
- 1/4 cup almond butter
- 1 tablespoon honey
- 1/4 cup unsweetened coconut flakes
- 1 tablespoon chia seeds

How to Prepare:

1. In a large mixing bowl, combine oats, almond butter, honey, coconut flakes, and chia seeds.
2. Stir the mixture until fully combined.
3. Roll the mixture into 12 small balls using your hands.
4. Refrigerate for 30 minutes to firm up.
5. Serve and enjoy!

Nutrition Facts (per serving):

- Calories: 150
- Protein: 4g
- Fat: 9g
- Carbs: 14g

72. Quinoa Salad Cups

Prep Time: 10 minutes
Cook Time: 15 minutes
Total Time: 25 minutes
Servings: 4
Yield: 4 servings

Ingredients:

- 1 cup cooked quinoa
- 1/2 cucumber, diced
- 1/2 avocado, diced
- 1 tablespoon olive oil
- 1 tablespoon chopped parsley

How to Prepare:

1. Cook quinoa according to package instructions and let it cool.
2. In a bowl, mix cooked quinoa, diced cucumber, avocado, and chopped parsley.
3. Drizzle olive oil on top and stir gently to combine.
4. Serve in individual cups.

Nutrition Facts (per serving):

- Calories: 180
- Protein: 5g
- Fat: 11g
- Carbs: 19g

73. Coconut Yogurt with Blueberries

Prep Time: 5 minutes
Cook Time: 0 minutes
Total Time: 5 minutes
Servings: 1
Yield: 1 serving

Ingredients:
- 1/2 cup unsweetened coconut yogurt
- 1/4 cup blueberries

How to Prepare:
1. In a bowl, add the coconut yogurt.
2. Top with fresh blueberries.
3. Serve immediately.

Nutrition Facts (per serving):
- Calories: 120
- Protein: 2g
- Fat: 9g
- Carbs: 14g

74. Cucumber and Avocado Slices

Prep Time: 5 minutes
Cook Time: 0 minutes
Total Time: 5 minutes
Servings: 1
Yield: 1 serving

Ingredients:
- 1/2 cucumber, sliced
- 1/2 avocado, sliced
- 1 tablespoon olive oil
- 1/4 teaspoon sea salt (optional)

How to Prepare:
1. Slice the cucumber and avocado.
2. Arrange the slices on a plate.
3. Drizzle olive oil over the top.
4. Sprinkle with sea salt, if desired.
5. Serve immediately.

Nutrition Facts (per serving):
- Calories: 160
- Protein: 3g
- Fat: 14g
- Carbs: 10g

75. Steamed Sweet Potato Slices

Prep Time: 5 minutes
Cook Time: 10 minutes
Total Time: 15 minutes
Servings: 2
Yield: 2 servings

Ingredients:

- 2 medium sweet potatoes, peeled and sliced
- 1 tablespoon olive oil
- 1/4 teaspoon cinnamon (optional)

How to Prepare:

1. Steam the sweet potato slices for about 10 minutes, or until soft.
2. Once steamed, drizzle with olive oil.
3. Sprinkle cinnamon (optional) for extra flavor.
4. Serve immediately.

Nutrition Facts (per serving):

- Calories: 150
- Protein: 2g
- Fat: 6g
- Carbs: 25g

76. Baked Sweet Potato Fries

Prep Time: 10 minutes
Cook Time: 30 minutes
Total Time: 40 minutes
Servings: 4
Yield: 4 servings

Ingredients:

- 2 medium sweet potatoes, cut into fries
- 1 tablespoon olive oil
- 1 teaspoon rosemary
- 1/4 teaspoon sea salt

How to Prepare:

1. Preheat the oven to 425°F (220°C).
2. Toss the sweet potato fries in olive oil, rosemary, and sea salt.
3. Spread the fries evenly on a baking sheet.
4. Bake for 25-30 minutes, flipping halfway through, until crispy and golden.
5. Serve immediately.

Nutrition Facts (per serving):

- Calories: 180
- Protein: 3g
- Fat: 7g
- Carbs: 30g

77. Peach Chia Smoothie

Prep Time: 5 minutes
Cook Time: 0 minutes
Total Time: 5 minutes
Servings: 2
Yield: 2 servings

Ingredients:
- 1 cup peaches, frozen
- 1 tablespoon chia seeds
- 1 cup coconut milk (unsweetened)

How to Prepare:
1. Combine the frozen peaches, chia seeds, and coconut milk in a blender.
2. Blend until smooth.
3. Serve chilled.

Nutrition Facts (per serving):
- Calories: 120
- Protein: 2g
- Fat: 7g
- Carbs: 14g

78. Hummus and Rice Crackers

Prep Time: 5 minutes
Cook Time: 0 minutes
Total Time: 5 minutes
Servings: 1
Yield: 1 serving

Ingredients:

- 1/4 cup homemade hummus (olive oil, tahini, garlic)
- 8 rice crackers

How to Prepare:

1. Serve hummus in a small dish.
2. Arrange rice crackers around the hummus.
3. Serve immediately.

Nutrition Facts (per serving):

- Calories: 180
- Protein: 5g
- Fat: 12g
- Carbs: 16g

79. Coconut Flake Energy Balls

Prep Time: 10 minutes
Cook Time: 0 minutes
Total Time: 10 minutes
Servings: 12 balls
Yield: 12 balls

Ingredients:
- 1/2 cup unsweetened coconut flakes
- 1/4 cup almond butter
- 1 cup oats
- 2 tablespoons honey
- 1 tablespoon chia seeds

How to Prepare:
1. In a large mixing bowl, combine coconut flakes, almond butter, oats, honey, and chia seeds.
2. Stir until fully combined.
3. Roll the mixture into 12 small balls.
4. Refrigerate for 30 minutes to firm up.
5. Serve and enjoy!

Nutrition Facts (per serving):
- Calories: 140
- Protein: 4g
- Fat: 10g
- Carbs: 12g

80. Avocado Smoothie

Prep Time: 5 minutes
Cook Time: 0 minutes
Total Time: 5 minutes
Servings: 1
Yield: 1 serving

Ingredients:
- 1/2 avocado
- 1 cup coconut milk (unsweetened)
- 1 teaspoon honey (optional)

How to Prepare:
1. Combine the avocado, coconut milk, and honey (if using) in a blender.
2. Blend until smooth.
3. Serve chilled.

Nutrition Facts (per serving):
- Calories: 190
- Protein: 2g
- Fat: 17g
- Carbs: 12g

Chapter 4: 14-Day Meal Plan for IC Patients

DAY 1

Breakfast: Banana and Almond Butter Bites

Ingredients: 1 banana, 2 tablespoons almond butter

Preparation: Slice banana into rounds, spread almond butter on each slice, and assemble the bites.

Macros: Calories: 180, Protein: 4g, Fat: 14g, Carbs: 16g

Lunch: Cucumber and Avocado Slices

Ingredients: 1/2 cucumber, 1/2 avocado, 1 tablespoon olive oil, sea salt (optional)

Preparation: Slice cucumber and avocado, arrange on a plate, drizzle with olive oil, and sprinkle with sea salt if desired.

Macros: Calories: 160, Protein: 3g, Fat: 14g, Carbs: 10g

Dinner: Baked Sweet Potato Fries

Ingredients: 2 medium sweet potatoes, 1 tablespoon olive oil, 1 teaspoon rosemary, sea salt

Preparation: Preheat oven to 425°F, toss sweet potato fries with olive oil, rosemary, and sea salt, and bake for 25-30 minutes.

Macros: Calories: 180, Protein: 3g, Fat: 7g, Carbs: 30g

Snack: Rice Cakes with Avocado

Ingredients: 2 rice cakes (plain), 1/2 avocado, 1 tablespoon olive oil, 1 tablespoon hemp seeds

Preparation: Top rice cakes with mashed avocado, drizzle with olive oil, and sprinkle with hemp seeds.

Macros: Calories: 220, Protein: 4g, Fat: 16g, Carbs: 20g

DAY 2

Breakfast: Oatmeal Energy Balls

Ingredients: 1 cup oats, 1/4 cup almond butter, 1 tablespoon honey, 1/4 cup unsweetened coconut flakes, 1 tablespoon chia seeds

Preparation: Mix all ingredients together, roll into 12 balls, refrigerate for 30 minutes.

Macros: Calories: 150, Protein: 4g, Fat: 9g, Carbs: 14g

Lunch: Quinoa Salad Cups

Ingredients: 1 cup cooked quinoa, 1/2 cucumber (diced), 1/2 avocado (diced), 1 tablespoon olive oil, 1 tablespoon parsley

Preparation: Combine quinoa, cucumber, avocado, parsley, and olive oil in a bowl, and serve in cups.

Macros: Calories: 180, Protein: 5g, Fat: 11g, Carbs: 19g

Dinner: Steamed Sweet Potato Slices

Ingredients: 2 sweet potatoes, 1 tablespoon olive oil, cinnamon (optional)

Preparation: Steam sweet potato slices for 10 minutes, drizzle with olive oil, and sprinkle with cinnamon if desired.

Macros: Calories: 150, Protein: 2g, Fat: 6g, Carbs: 25g

Snack: Coconut Chia Pudding

Ingredients: 2 tablespoons chia seeds, 1 cup unsweetened coconut milk, 1 teaspoon honey (optional)

Preparation: Mix chia seeds and coconut milk, refrigerate for 4 hours or overnight, and top with honey if desired.

Macros: Calories: 180, Protein: 4g, Fat: 14g, Carbs: 14g

DAY 3

Breakfast: Non-Dairy Yogurt Parfait

Ingredients: 1/2 cup unsweetened almond milk yogurt, 1/4 cup blueberries, 2 tablespoons oats, 1 tablespoon chia seeds

Preparation: Layer yogurt, blueberries, oats, and chia seeds in a glass or bowl.

Macros: Calories: 150, Protein: 4g, Fat: 6g, Carbs: 20g

Lunch: Rice Cake with Almond Butter and Pear Slices

Ingredients: 2 rice cakes (plain), 2 tablespoons almond butter, 1 pear (sliced)

Preparation: Spread almond butter on rice cakes, top with pear slices, and serve.

Macros: Calories: 220, Protein: 5g, Fat: 14g, Carbs: 25g

Dinner: Coconut Yogurt with Blueberries

Ingredients: 1/2 cup unsweetened coconut yogurt, 1/4 cup blueberries

Preparation: Combine coconut yogurt and blueberries in a bowl and serve.

Macros: Calories: 120, Protein: 2g, Fat: 9g, Carbs: 14g

Snack: Banana and Almond Butter Bites

Ingredients: 1 banana, 2 tablespoons almond butter

Preparation: Slice banana into rounds, spread almond butter on each slice, and assemble the bites.

Macros: Calories: 180, Protein: 4g, Fat: 14g, Carbs: 16g

DAY 4

Breakfast: Zucchini Chips

Ingredients: 2 zucchinis, 1 tablespoon olive oil, sea salt (optional)

Preparation: Slice zucchinis thinly, toss with olive oil and salt, and bake at 375°F for 20 minutes.

Macros: Calories: 120, Protein: 2g, Fat: 9g, Carbs: 15g

Lunch: Carrot and Cucumber Sticks with Hummus

Ingredients: 2 carrots, 1 cucumber, 1/4 cup homemade hummus (olive oil, tahini, garlic)

Preparation: Slice carrots and cucumber into sticks, serve with hummus.

Macros: Calories: 180, Protein: 5g, Fat: 12g, Carbs: 20g

Dinner: Baked Sweet Potato Fries

Ingredients: 2 sweet potatoes, 1 tablespoon olive oil, 1 teaspoon rosemary, sea salt

Preparation: Preheat oven to 425°F, toss sweet potato fries with olive oil, rosemary, and sea salt, and bake for 25-30 minutes.

Macros: Calories: 180, Protein: 3g, Fat: 7g, Carbs: 30g

Snack: Coconut Flake Energy Balls

Ingredients: 1/2 cup unsweetened coconut flakes, 1/4 cup almond butter, 1 cup oats, 2 tablespoons honey, 1 tablespoon chia seeds

Preparation: Mix all ingredients, roll into balls, and refrigerate for 30 minutes.

Macros: Calories: 140, Protein: 4g, Fat: 10g, Carbs: 12g

DAY 5

Breakfast: Peach Chia Smoothie

Ingredients: 1 cup frozen peaches, 1 tablespoon chia seeds, 1 cup coconut milk (unsweetened)

Preparation: Blend peaches, chia seeds, and coconut milk until smooth.

Macros: Calories: 120, Protein: 2g, Fat: 7g, Carbs: 14g

Lunch: Avocado Smoothie

Ingredients: 1/2 avocado, 1 cup coconut milk (unsweetened), 1 teaspoon honey (optional)

Preparation: Blend avocado, coconut milk, and honey until smooth.

Macros: Calories: 190, Protein: 2g, Fat: 17g, Carbs: 12g

Dinner: Quinoa Salad Cups

Ingredients: 1 cup cooked quinoa, 1/2 cucumber (diced), 1/2 avocado (diced), 1 tablespoon olive oil, 1 tablespoon parsley

Preparation: Combine quinoa, cucumber, avocado, parsley, and olive oil in a bowl, and serve in cups.

Macros: Calories: 180, Protein: 5g, Fat: 11g, Carbs: 19g

Snack: Apple Slices with Almond Butter

Ingredients: 1 apple, 2 tablespoons almond butter

Preparation: Slice apple and serve with almond butter.

Macros: Calories: 200, Protein: 4g, Fat: 16g, Carbs: 24g

DAY 6

Breakfast: Homemade Granola Bars

Ingredients: 1 cup oats, 2 tablespoons honey, 1/4 cup mild fruits (e.g. pears), 1/4 cup unsweetened coconut flakes, 1 tablespoon chia seeds, 2 tablespoons almond butter

Preparation: Mix all ingredients, press into a baking dish, refrigerate until firm.

Macros: Calories: 180, Protein: 4g, Fat: 9g, Carbs: 21g

Lunch: Cucumber and Avocado Slices

Ingredients: 1/2 cucumber, 1/2 avocado, 1 tablespoon olive oil, sea salt (optional)

Preparation: Slice cucumber and avocado, arrange on a plate, drizzle with olive oil, and sprinkle with sea salt if desired.

Macros: Calories: 160, Protein: 3g, Fat: 14g, Carbs: 10g

Dinner: Steamed Sweet Potato Slices

Ingredients: 2 medium sweet potatoes, 1 tablespoon olive oil, cinnamon (optional)

Preparation: Steam sweet potato slices for 10 minutes, drizzle with olive oil, and sprinkle with cinnamon if desired.

Macros: Calories: 150, Protein: 2g, Fat: 6g, Carbs: 25g

Snack: Hummus and Rice Crackers

Ingredients: 1/4 cup homemade hummus (olive oil, tahini), 8 rice crackers

Preparation: Serve hummus with rice crackers.

Macros: Calories: 180, Protein: 5g, Fat: 12g, Carbs: 16g

DAY 7

Breakfast: Coconut Chia Pudding

Ingredients: 2 tablespoons chia seeds, 1 cup unsweetened coconut milk, 1 teaspoon honey (optional)

Preparation: Mix chia seeds and coconut milk, refrigerate for 4 hours or overnight, and top with honey if desired.

Macros: Calories: 180, Protein: 4g, Fat: 14g, Carbs: 14g

Lunch: Rice Cakes with Avocado

Ingredients: 2 rice cakes (plain), 1/2 avocado, 1 tablespoon olive oil, 1 tablespoon hemp seeds

Preparation: Top rice cakes with mashed avocado, drizzle with olive oil, and sprinkle with hemp seeds.

Macros: Calories: 220, Protein: 4g, Fat: 16g, Carbs: 20g

Dinner: Baked Apple Chips

Ingredients: 2 apples, cinnamon (optional)

Preparation: Slice apples thinly, place on a baking sheet, and bake at 200°F for 1-1.5 hours until crisp.

Macros: Calories: 120, Protein: 1g, Fat: 0g, Carbs: 32g

Snack: Zucchini Chips

Ingredients: 2 zucchinis, 1 tablespoon olive oil, sea salt (optional)

Preparation: Slice zucchinis thinly, toss with olive oil and salt, and bake at 375°F for 20 minutes.

Macros: Calories: 120, Protein: 2g, Fat: 9g, Carbs: 15g

DAY 8

Breakfast: Oatmeal Energy Balls

Ingredients: 1 cup oats, 1/4 cup almond butter, 1 tablespoon honey, 1/4 cup unsweetened coconut flakes, 1 tablespoon chia seeds

Preparation: Mix all ingredients together, roll into 12 balls, refrigerate for 30 minutes.

Macros: Calories: 150, Protein: 4g, Fat: 9g, Carbs: 14g

Lunch: Carrot and Cucumber Sticks with Hummus

Ingredients: 2 carrots, 1 cucumber, 1/4 cup homemade hummus (olive oil, tahini, garlic)

Preparation: Slice carrots and cucumber into sticks, serve with hummus.

Macros: Calories: 180, Protein: 5g, Fat: 12g, Carbs: 20g

Dinner: Quinoa Salad Cups

Ingredients: 1 cup cooked quinoa, 1/2 cucumber (diced), 1/2 avocado (diced), 1 tablespoon olive oil, 1 tablespoon parsley

Preparation: Combine quinoa, cucumber, avocado, parsley, and olive oil in a bowl, and serve in cups.

Macros: Calories: 180, Protein: 5g, Fat: 11g, Carbs: 19g

Snack: Banana and Almond Butter Bites

Ingredients: 1 banana, 2 tablespoons almond butter

Preparation: Slice banana into rounds, spread almond butter on each slice, and assemble the bites.

Macros: Calories: 180, Protein: 4g, Fat: 14g, Carbs: 16g

DAY 9

Breakfast: Rice Cake with Almond Butter and Pear Slices

Ingredients: 2 rice cakes (plain), 2 tablespoons almond butter, 1 pear (sliced)

Preparation: Spread almond butter on rice cakes, top with pear slices, and serve.

Macros: Calories: 220, Protein: 5g, Fat: 14g, Carbs: 25g

Lunch: Cucumber and Avocado Slices

Ingredients: 1/2 cucumber, 1/2 avocado, 1 tablespoon olive oil, sea salt (optional)

Preparation: Slice cucumber and avocado, arrange on a plate, drizzle with olive oil, and sprinkle with sea salt if desired.

Macros: Calories: 160, Protein: 3g, Fat: 14g, Carbs: 10g

Dinner: Steamed Sweet Potato Slices

Ingredients: 2 medium sweet potatoes, 1 tablespoon olive oil, cinnamon (optional)

Preparation: Steam sweet potato slices for 10 minutes, drizzle with olive oil, and sprinkle with cinnamon if desired.

Macros: Calories: 150, Protein: 2g, Fat: 6g, Carbs: 25g

Snack: Coconut Flake Energy Balls

Ingredients: 1/2 cup unsweetened coconut flakes, 1/4 cup almond butter, 1 cup oats, 2 tablespoons honey, 1 tablespoon chia seeds

Preparation: Mix all ingredients, roll into balls, and refrigerate for 30 minutes.

Macros: Calories: 140, Protein: 4g, Fat: 10g, Carbs: 12g

DAY 10

Breakfast: Peach Chia Smoothie

Ingredients: 1 cup frozen peaches, 1 tablespoon chia seeds, 1 cup coconut milk (unsweetened)

Preparation: Blend peaches, chia seeds, and coconut milk until smooth.

Macros: Calories: 120, Protein: 2g, Fat: 7g, Carbs: 14g

Lunch: Hummus and Rice Crackers

Ingredients: 1/4 cup homemade hummus (olive oil, tahini), 8 rice crackers

Preparation: Serve hummus with rice crackers.

Macros: Calories: 180, Protein: 5g, Fat: 12g, Carbs: 16g

Dinner: Baked Apple Chips

Ingredients: 2 apples, cinnamon (optional)

Preparation: Slice apples thinly, place on a baking sheet, and bake at 200°F for 1-1.5 hours until crisp.

Macros: Calories: 120, Protein: 1g, Fat: 0g, Carbs: 32g

Snack: Avocado Smoothie

Ingredients: 1/2 avocado, 1 cup coconut milk (unsweetened), 1 teaspoon honey (optional)

Preparation: Blend avocado, coconut milk, and honey until smooth.

Macros: Calories: 190, Protein: 2g, Fat: 17g, Carbs: 12g

DAY 11

Breakfast: Non-Dairy Yogurt Parfait

Ingredients: 1/2 cup unsweetened almond milk yogurt, 1/4 cup blueberries, 2 tablespoons oats, 1 tablespoon chia seeds

Preparation: Layer yogurt, blueberries, oats, and chia seeds in a glass or bowl.

Macros: Calories: 150, Protein: 4g, Fat: 6g, Carbs: 20g

Lunch: Cucumber and Avocado Slices

Ingredients: 1/2 cucumber, 1/2 avocado, 1 tablespoon olive oil, sea salt (optional)

Preparation: Slice cucumber and avocado, arrange on a plate, drizzle with olive oil, and sprinkle with sea salt if desired.

Macros: Calories: 160, Protein: 3g, Fat: 14g, Carbs: 10g

Dinner: Baked Sweet Potato Fries

Ingredients: 2 medium sweet potatoes, 1 tablespoon olive oil, 1 teaspoon rosemary, sea salt

Preparation: Preheat oven to 425°F, toss sweet potato fries with olive oil, rosemary, and sea salt, and bake for 25-30 minutes.

Macros: Calories: 180, Protein: 3g, Fat: 7g, Carbs: 30g

Snack: Zucchini Chips

Ingredients: 2 zucchinis, 1 tablespoon olive oil, sea salt (optional)

Preparation: Slice zucchinis thinly, toss with olive oil and salt, and bake at 375°F for 20 minutes.

Macros: Calories: 120, Protein: 2g, Fat: 9g, Carbs: 15g

DAY 12

Breakfast: Oatmeal Energy Balls

Ingredients: 1 cup oats, 1/4 cup almond butter, 1 tablespoon honey, 1/4 cup unsweetened coconut flakes, 1 tablespoon chia seeds

Preparation: Mix all ingredients together, roll into 12 balls, refrigerate for 30 minutes.

Macros: Calories: 150, Protein: 4g, Fat: 9g, Carbs: 14g

Lunch: Rice Cake with Almond Butter and Pear Slices

Ingredients: 2 rice cakes (plain), 2 tablespoons almond butter, 1 pear (sliced)

Preparation: Spread almond butter on rice cakes, top with pear slices, and serve.

Macros: Calories: 220, Protein: 5g, Fat: 14g, Carbs: 25g

Dinner: Steamed Sweet Potato Slices

Ingredients: 2 medium sweet potatoes, 1 tablespoon olive oil, cinnamon (optional)

Preparation: Steam sweet potato slices for 10 minutes, drizzle with olive oil, and sprinkle with cinnamon if desired.

Macros: Calories: 150, Protein: 2g, Fat: 6g, Carbs: 25g

Snack: Coconut Flake Energy Balls

Ingredients: 1/2 cup unsweetened coconut flakes, 1/4 cup almond butter, 1 cup oats, 2 tablespoons honey, 1 tablespoon chia seeds

Preparation: Mix all ingredients, roll into balls, and refrigerate for 30 minutes.

Macros: Calories: 140, Protein: 4g, Fat: 10g, Carbs: 12g

DAY 13

Breakfast: Peach Chia Smoothie

Ingredients: 1 cup frozen peaches, 1 tablespoon chia seeds, 1 cup coconut milk (unsweetened)

Preparation: Blend peaches, chia seeds, and coconut milk until smooth.

Macros: Calories: 120, Protein: 2g, Fat: 7g, Carbs: 14g

Lunch: Cucumber and Avocado Slices

Ingredients: 1/2 cucumber, 1/2 avocado, 1 tablespoon olive oil, sea salt (optional)

Preparation: Slice cucumber and avocado, arrange on a plate, drizzle with olive oil, and sprinkle with sea salt if desired.

Macros: Calories: 160, Protein: 3g, Fat: 14g, Carbs: 10g

Dinner: Baked Apple Chips

Ingredients: 2 apples, cinnamon (optional)

Preparation: Slice apples thinly, place on a baking sheet, and bake at 200°F for 1-1.5 hours until crisp.

Macros: Calories: 120, Protein: 1g, Fat: 0g, Carbs: 32g

Snack: Rice Cakes with Avocado

Ingredients: 2 rice cakes (plain), 1/2 avocado, 1 tablespoon olive oil, 1 tablespoon hemp seeds

Preparation: Top rice cakes with mashed avocado, drizzle with olive oil, and sprinkle with hemp seeds.

Macros: Calories: 220, Protein: 4g, Fat: 16g, Carbs: 20g

DAY 14

Breakfast: Homemade Granola Bars

Ingredients: 1 cup oats, 2 tablespoons honey, 1/4 cup mild fruits (e.g., pears), 1/4 cup unsweetened coconut flakes, 1 tablespoon chia seeds, 2 tablespoons almond butter

Preparation: Mix all ingredients, press into a baking dish, refrigerate until firm.

Macros: Calories: 180, Protein: 4g, Fat: 9g, Carbs: 21g

Lunch: Avocado Smoothie

Ingredients: 1/2 avocado, 1 cup coconut milk (unsweetened), 1 teaspoon honey (optional)

Preparation: Blend avocado, coconut milk, and honey until smooth.

Macros: Calories: 190, Protein: 2g, Fat: 17g, Carbs: 12g

Dinner: Coconut Yogurt with Blueberries

Ingredients: 1/2 cup unsweetened coconut yogurt, 1/4 cup blueberries

Preparation: Combine coconut yogurt and blueberries in a bowl and serve.

Macros: Calories: 120, Protein: 2g, Fat: 9g, Carbs: 14g

Snack: Banana and Almond Butter Bites

Ingredients: 1 banana, 2 tablespoons almond butter

Preparation: Slice banana into rounds, spread almond butter on each slice, and assemble the bites.

Macros: Calories: 180, Protein: 4g, Fat: 14g, Carbs: 16g

Chapter 5: Caring for a Loved One with IC — Practical Support for Family Members and Caregivers

Helping with Food Choices and Meal Prep for Someone Living with Interstitial Cystitis

Caring for someone with Interstitial Cystitis (IC) means being there not only physically but also emotionally. As your loved one manages their dietary limitations, your involvement can be a huge source of relief. Caregivers have the power to make meals feel less stressful, more manageable, and even enjoyable. Here are some helpful and meaningful ways you can support someone with IC through smart food choices and thoughtful meal preparation:

1. Learn About Foods That Help—and Those That Hurt

To give the best support, it's important to know which foods are bladder-friendly and which ones commonly cause flare-ups. Things like citrus fruits, tomatoes, chocolate, spicy dishes, and alcohol are often irritating and should be avoided. Instead, focus on simple, calming, and anti-inflammatory foods like oats, rice, lean meats, avocado, and gentle fruits such as apples and pears. Work closely with your loved one to build meals around these IC-friendly options, so they always feel safe and supported when it's time to eat.

2. Plan and Prep Meals Together

Meal planning is one of the best ways to reduce stress and avoid last-minute food choices that might trigger symptoms. Helping with meal prep—like cooking together or organizing meals in advance—can be a major help. Try batch cooking: preparing larger portions of safe meals that can be portioned out and stored for the next few days. Use containers to keep servings separate and easy to reheat. This keeps nutritious, IC-safe food easily accessible and minimizes the need for rushed decisions.

3. Make Mealtimes Calm and Comfortable

Creating a peaceful, pleasant atmosphere during meals can make a big difference. The emotional state of someone living with IC can influence their symptoms, so a relaxed, reassuring mealtime setting is beneficial. Don't rush through meals—give plenty of time for eating slowly and peacefully, as stress or hurried eating can disrupt digestion and potentially trigger discomfort. Small touches like soft lighting or a favorite playlist can also add comfort.

4. Keep Meals Fun and Flavorful

Following a restricted diet doesn't mean food has to be boring! Help your loved one explore exciting, creative meals using safe ingredients. Try new IC-friendly recipes or come up with unique twists using familiar ingredients—like swapping pasta for spiralized zucchini or blending up a smoothie with pears, rice milk, and chia seeds. Making meals exciting can lift their spirits and keep them engaged with their dietary needs in a positive way.

5. Be Understanding When Symptoms Flare

Even with careful planning, there will be days when symptoms flare up. This isn't anyone's fault—factors like stress, lack of sleep, or unknown triggers can cause bad days. On these days, show patience and compassion. Offer help without pressure and be gentle, both emotionally and physically. Sometimes, just sitting with them or bringing a heating pad is the most valuable thing you can do.

6. Focus on Balance and Nutrition

Eating a well-rounded diet is just as important for someone with IC as it is for anyone else—it just takes a bit more care. Support your loved one in getting enough essential nutrients without triggering their symptoms. Help make sure they're getting healthy fats (like olive oil or avocado), quality proteins (like tofu or chicken), and fiber-rich foods (like oats, veggies, or quinoa). This helps them feel strong and nourished, and may also help their body better manage symptoms over time.

7. Be Extra Supportive During Flare-Ups

When a flare-up hits, your loved one might need extra help with food and comfort. Stick to simple, soothing foods—plain rice, cooked carrots, or boiled potatoes often work well. Don't force them to eat if their appetite is low. Instead, gently encourage hydration with safe fluids like filtered water or calming teas such as chamomile or ginger. These small gestures can offer physical comfort and show deep emotional care.

8. Be There Emotionally—It Matters More Than You Know

Living with a chronic condition like IC can take an emotional toll. Your role as a caregiver isn't just about food or errands—it's also about listening with kindness, showing empathy, and reminding them they're not alone. Let them vent, cry, or share without trying to "fix" everything. Sometimes, being a steady and understanding presence is the most healing kind of support you can offer.

It's good to know that caring for someone with IC may come with challenges, but your efforts—big or small—can create a safer, more comforting daily life for your loved one. From meal prep to moral support, you're not just helping them eat better—you're helping them live better.

Dining Out and Social Gatherings: How to Navigate Restaurants and Events While Following the IC Diet

Managing interstitial cystitis (IC) while attending social functions or dining out can be a real challenge, especially when trying to stay loyal to a bladder-friendly diet that avoids common triggers. Still, with some strategic preparation and open communication, it's absolutely possible to enjoy these outings without compromising health. Here are some practical and supportive tips for caregivers and family members to help navigate these experiences with ease:

1. Call Restaurants in Advance

Before heading out to eat, take a few minutes to call the restaurant and explain your loved one's dietary restrictions. These days, many restaurants are more aware and accommodating of special dietary needs. Ask whether they can prepare meals with mild, simple ingredients—think steamed veggies, plain chicken, or plain rice. Giving the kitchen a heads-up often allows for easier customizations than trying to make last-minute requests at the table.

2. Know the Bladder-Friendly Choices

When reviewing a menu, it's helpful to already know which foods are safer for those with IC. Choose dishes that are steamed, grilled, or roasted with minimal seasoning. Grilled chicken or fish, roasted sweet potatoes, and plain rice are solid options. Avoid spicy meals, acidic sauces, or anything containing tomato, citrus, or caffeine, which are common IC triggers.

3. Bring Your Own Safe Snacks

For social events or parties where food choices may not be IC-safe, consider preparing and bringing your own snacks or dishes. Homemade granola bars, rice cakes with almond butter, fresh apples or pears, or baked sweet potato fries are great options. Having safe food on hand ensures your loved one won't feel excluded or hungry while others are eating.

4. Shift Focus Away from Food

Socializing doesn't always need to revolve around eating. Suggest events or outings that highlight fun, food-free activities—like going for a walk, catching a movie, or visiting a museum. When attention is shifted to entertainment or company rather than food, the experience becomes more inclusive and enjoyable for everyone.

5. Carry IC-Friendly Beverages

If drinks are a concern, bring a bladder-safe beverage along. A reusable water bottle filled with filtered water, chamomile or ginger tea, or cucumber-mint infused water are great options. These help keep your loved one hydrated without irritating the bladder. At events, gracefully decline caffeinated or alcoholic drinks and explain if needed why those are off-limits.

6. Speak Up About Dietary Needs

Don't hesitate to be honest and advocate for your loved one's dietary needs when attending gatherings. Politely informing hosts or restaurant staff about restrictions can go a long way. Most people will appreciate the transparency and want to help by offering safe food options.

7. Use the Moment to Educate Others

If your loved one is comfortable, consider using social occasions as a chance to spread awareness about IC and its dietary implications. This not only helps friends and family understand the condition but also fosters a more supportive and empathetic environment, making future events easier and more welcoming.

8. Choose Smaller Portions When Unsure

When it's unclear what's in a dish or whether it's IC-friendly, encourage your loved one to try just a small portion. Sampling in moderation reduces the chance of triggering symptoms and helps them avoid a full flare-up if something doesn't agree with their system.

9. Stay Positive and Calm

It's natural to feel frustrated about missing out on certain foods during social events, but maintaining a calm, upbeat attitude makes a big difference. As a caregiver, modeling resilience and optimism can help your loved one stay positive too. Focus on enjoying the moment, the people, and the fun rather than just the food.

10. Plan Ahead for Special Occasions

Celebrations like birthdays or holidays are easier to manage with a little planning. Ensure that IC-friendly dishes are included in the spread and offer to bring a safe, tasty dish your loved one can eat without worry. These events don't need to center around problematic foods—with preparation, everyone can enjoy the occasion together comfortably.

Conclusion

Managing the day-to-day realities of living with Interstitial Cystitis (IC) requires more than just dietary changes—it involves creating a nurturing and informed approach to daily living that prioritizes comfort, wellness, and understanding. By recognizing the crucial role that food, hydration, and lifestyle choices play in symptom control, both caregivers and patients can build a solid foundation for living well with IC. A collaborative and compassionate approach to meal planning and self-care helps reduce flare-ups while also providing physical and emotional support.

Following an IC-friendly diet means choosing foods that are both gentle on the bladder and packed with nutritional value. Avoiding acidic fruits, caffeine, spicy ingredients, and other known irritants is essential, but so is embracing meals that soothe and nourish. Simple, home-cooked foods made with safe, healing ingredients can make a meaningful difference. Planning meals ahead of time allows caregivers and family members to feel confident that their loved one is eating in a way that supports their body—without the stress of making last-minute choices that could lead to discomfort.

The involvement of family members and caregivers is a cornerstone of successfully managing IC. Your support can have a powerful effect—whether it's preparing meals that won't trigger symptoms, offering a listening ear during challenging moments, or simply learning more about the condition to provide better care. Knowing which foods are safe and understanding the importance of dietary boundaries allows caregivers to protect their loved one's health while still helping them feel included and supported.

Though IC presents real and ongoing challenges, it doesn't have to stand in the way of a joyful and balanced lifestyle. With the right tools, preparation, and awareness, those living with IC can still enjoy their meals, relationships, and daily routines. Embracing the guidelines of the IC diet, staying vigilant about potential triggers, and offering consistent emotional and practical support can empower patients to feel more in control and less burdened by their condition.

In the end, thriving with IC is entirely possible when there is a strong support system in place. Patients and caregivers, working together, can cultivate a lifestyle filled with thoughtful choices, loving care, and shared understanding—ensuring that each day is met with comfort, connection, and a sense of wellbeing.

Printed in Great Britain
by Amazon